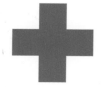

Canadian Red Cross

Child Care
First Aid & CPR
Manual

This manual belongs to:

_____

StayWell

StayWell

Cette publication est disponible en français.

The terms he and she have been used throughout the manual to ensure representation of both genders and to correspond to any photos within a particular section.

Composition by Embassy Graphics
Printing/binding by Printcrafters Inc.

Printed in Canada by:
The StayWell Health Company Ltd.
2 Quebec Street, Suite 107, Guelph ON N1H 2T3
A division of
StayWell
780 Township Line Road, Yardley, PA 19067-4200 USA

ISBN 10 : 1-58480-350-9
ISBN 13 : 978-1-58480-350-8

09 10 11 / 6 5 4

Contents

Acknowledgements

The Canadian Red Cross Child Care program was developed by combining the National ChildSafe program and the Western Canadian Child Care First Aid Program, which have been developed over the past 18 years. Each time the program undergoes a revision, it starts with a foundation of the great work completed in the previous revision. We would like to recognize everyone who worked on the programs and products before us.

This revision is dedicated to the memory of Karen Shank, who helped lay the foundation for managing this project.

This project was completed because of the creative vision, ongoing support and dedication of the team at our publishing partner StayWell, the Project Executive Sponsor: Yvan Chalifour, National Director, Injury Prevention; Project Sponsor: Rick Caissie, National Manager First Aid; Project Manager: Cathy Forner, National Project Management Officer, Injury Prevention; and ECC Canada Liaison and Technical Advisor: Tracey Braun, National First Aid Coordinator.

The **Primary Project Team** was responsible for providing the overall leadership and direction for the project and was made up of: Kelly Ducharme, National Marketing and Promotions Officer; Colleen Lavender, National Marketing and Promotions Officer; Laura McNamara, First Aid Injury Prevention Advisor, Atlantic Zone; Tannis Nostedt, First Aid Program Advisor; Western Zone, Elizabeth Ramlogan, First Aid Services, Program Advisor, Ontario Zone; Eric Ritterrath, National Coordinator, Publications; Sylvie Santerre, Senior Coordinator, Injury Prevention Services, Quebec Zone; Janel Swain, National Project Technical Advisor; and Carolyn Tees, National Marketing and Business Development Officer.

The Canadian Red Cross **National Medical Advisory Team** reviewed the content of the program and was made up of: Brendan J. Hughes MD, CCFP; Andrew MacPherson BSc, MD, CCFP-EM, Chief, Department of Emergency Medicine, Vancouver Island Health Authority, Victoria; and Ernest Prégent MD CCFP(em) CSPQ, FCCFP

External review, guidance and endorsement of the program content was thanks to: Kim Tytler - Canadian Child Care Federation, and Peter O'Neil, Smart Risk

There was excellent market research which guided the project's direction and vision. We would like to thank the many Authorized Providers, Instructor Trainers, and Instructors who participated in the market research. Their input and guidance helped shaped the new look of our programs and products. The **Marketing Project Team** was responsible for marketing expertise and direction for the project and was provided by: Francoise Filteau, Senior Coordinator, Injury Prevention Services, Quebec Zone; Sue Phillips, Director First Aid and Water Safety, Western Zone; and Joan Savoie, Program Representative, Ontario Zone. A Marketing Advisory Panel supported the work of the Marketing Team and we would like to thank the 25 Authorized Providers, Instructors and Instructor Trainers from across Canada that provided their thoughts, advice and direction.

Child Care Sub-Committee Members - Karen Clark, British Columbia; Lorraine Cochrane, New Brunswick; Dominique Graf, Alberta; Brooke Hendricks, Alberta; Kevin Holder, Manitoba; Angela Moffat, Alberta; Megan Moffat, Alberta; and Lyne Tétreault, Quebec.

Reviewers and Contributors

Ethne Dickinson, Alberta; Anne Lacroix, Quebec; Johane Lafleur, Quebec; Nancy Reynolds, Quebec; Sarah Smith, British Columbia; Lisa Smith, Saskatchewan; and Charna VanEden, Alberta.

The Red Cross

The year is 1859. You are a soldier in the French army, and you have been severely wounded. As blood spurts out from a bullet hole in your thigh, you collapse onto the battlefield. You assume that you will die. Later, however, you find yourself confused but alive, lying next to an enemy soldier from the Austrian army. You are no longer on the battlefield, and strangers are tending to the wounds of yourself, your comrades, and your enemies. You are too grateful to be alive to think about war any longer.

HENRY DUNANT – The Red Cross Founder

- In June 1859, Henry Dunant (Figure 1.1) saw an unforgettable scene: 40,000 dead and wounded soldiers left on the field after the Battle of Solferino in Italy.

- Dunant organized local villagers into first aid teams to help as many of the wounded as possible, saving thousands of lives.

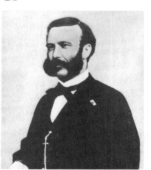

Figure 1.1 Henry Dunant.

> **NOTE:**
>
> *In December of 2005, the International Red Cross and Red Crescent Movement welcomed the decision to create an additional emblem alongside the red cross and red crescent, the red crystal.*

- To prevent this horror from happening again, he decided to create a neutral organization to care for wounded soldiers and prisoners—an organization that would be respected and protected by both sides in any conflict. The result was the Red Cross.

- Dunant spent the rest of his life trying to reduce the suffering caused by war. He lobbied governments, organized Red Cross Societies in different countries, and spoke to the public.

- Today, the symbol chosen for the Red Cross is recognized around the world: a red cross on a white background.

- In 1901, Dunant won the first Nobel Peace Prize. By founding the International Red Cross and Red Crescent Movement, he saved the lives of millions of people over the years.

- Red Cross first aid services, volunteer services, and family links were all started by Henry Dunant.

RED CROSS – Fundamental Principles

There are Red Cross or Red Crescent Societies in over 180 countries around the world.

In every country, our programs and activities are guided by seven Fundamental Principles. The Tanzanian Red Cross has created a short, simple version of these principles:

Humanity: We serve people, but not systems.

Impartiality: We care for the victims and the aggressors alike.

Neutrality: We take initiatives, but never take sides.

Independence: We bow to needs, but not rulers.

Voluntary Service: We work around the clock, but never for personal gain.

Unity: We have many talents, but a single idea.

Universality: We respect nations, but our work knows no bounds.

Essentially, we provide help to people in need, whatever their race, political beliefs, religion, social status, or culture.

WHO WE ARE – The Canadian Red Cross

Our Mission

The Canadian Red Cross mission is to improve the lives of vulnerable people by mobilizing the power of humanity in Canada and around the world.

Our Values

Our actions and decisions will be based upon:

- Humanitarian values, as expressed in our Fundamental Principles;
- Respect, dignity, and care for one another within and outside Red Cross; and
- Integrity, accountability, effectiveness, and transparency.

How We Help

Disaster Services

The Canadian Red Cross helps people affected by emergencies and disasters—situations ranging from a house fire to a flood that disrupts an entire region of the country.

International Programs

The Canadian Red Cross works in other countries to help people who have been affected by war and natural disasters to bring urgently needed relief items, reunite families, and help rebuild communities.

Family Links

The Canadian Red Cross helps reunite families who have lost touch as a result of war or natural disaster.

First Aid Programs

The Canadian Red Cross First Aid Program has been training Canadians in first aid for more than 50 years. Our courses give people the knowledge and skills to deal with emergency situations and to prevent injuries from happening.

Water Safety Services

Thanks to the work of Water Safety Services, more than 27 million Canadians have learned how to swim and safely enjoy water activities since 1946.

RespectED: Violence and Abuse Prevention

RespectED: Violence and Abuse Prevention programs promote safe and supportive relationships and healthy communities through education and partnerships.

Homecare Services

For more than 70 years, the Canadian Red Cross has been providing in-home community services to help individuals live as independently as possible.

Health Equipment Loan Programs

For more than 50 years, the Canadian Red Cross has been offering Health Equipment Loan Programs.

For further information on Canadian Red Cross services, visit our Website at www.redcross.ca.

Preparing to Respond

You have five young children in your care and, one afternoon, while they're playing a circle game on the floor, a four-year-old girl starts feeling ill and begins vomiting. You rush to assist her…

This manual focusses on how to provide first aid and safe environments for children. Many of the principles are the same as those for adults. Note carefully, however, the special comments about children. They apply to all caregivers, for example, parents, guardians, babysitters, and child care practitioners working in centres or family child care.

First aid is the immediate care you give to an ill or injured person until more advanced care can be obtained. Everyone should know first aid and know what to do in an emergency.

A **First Aider** is someone like you who has taken a first aid course. A First Aider can recognize a medical emergency and help those in need.

THE FIRST AIDER'S ROLE

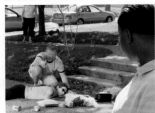

Your role includes three basic steps:

1. Recognize the emergency and act accordingly.
2. Call EMS/9-1-1 (Figure 2.1).
3. Act according to your skills, knowledge, and comfort level.

Figure 2.1 Calling EMS/ 9-1-1.

Firefighters, police, and ambulance personnel are people who may arrive on the scene of an emergency. But it always takes some time for them to arrive. Therefore, a First Aider already at the scene should help.

RECOGNIZING EMERGENCIES

The first step in dealing with an emergency is to recognize that it is an emergency.

• A **medical emergency** is an illness or condition that needs immediate medical attention. For example, an asthma attack is a medical emergency.

- An **injury** is some kind of damage to the body. This damage can include broken bones, wounds, and burns. The most common causes of injuries include motor vehicle collisions, falls, poisoning, and drowning. Some injuries are serious enough to be considered emergencies. If you're not sure, call EMS/9-1-1 and let the professionals decide.

PREPARE! STAY SAFE! SURVIVE!

- **Prepare!** includes everything you do before you start an activity, including taking a first aid course.
- **Stay Safe!** includes everything you do during the activity, such as wearing safety gear.
- **Survive!** includes actions you take to ensure the safety and survival of yourself and others, such as providing first aid in an emergency.

> **REMEMBER:**
>
> *Injuries are not accidents. Injuries are predictable and preventable. Planning for safety is the best way to prevent injuries.*
> *Good First Aiders keep safe and make wise choices. They help teach children about keeping safe and making wise choises as well.*

DECIDE TO ACT

Many lives are saved because people like you get involved. Every year, thousands of bystanders in Canada recognize and respond to emergencies. Some phone for help, some comfort the ill or injured person or family members, some give first aid, and some help keep order at the emergency scene.

Sometimes people don't want to get involved in an emergency, and this can be for various reasons. The five most common concerns are:

Other people at the scene: If there are other people at the scene, it may be easy to think that they will take care of the emergency without your help. However, you should never assume that someone is providing first aid just because you see many people around. And remember that there are many important jobs you can do: help control the crowd, call EMS/9-1-1, get supplies, or comfort the ill or injured person.

The ill or injured person: You may not feel comfortable treating an ill or injured person if he or she is behaving oddly, much older or younger than you, or of a different race or gender. Remember, whoever the person is, he or she needs help.

Unpleasant injuries or illnesses: You may feel upset or sick when you see blood, vomit, broken bones, or other injuries. If this happens, take a moment to calm down before you deal with the situation.

Catching a disease: You might be afraid that you could catch something from the injured person. There are many ways to reduce the risks, and we'll talk about them in this chapter.

Doing something wrong: You might be afraid of getting sued if you make a mistake. But as long as you act reasonably and carefully, you don't need to worry. Most provinces and territories have laws that protect bystanders who give emergency help. Just use common sense and don't try to do something you're not trained to do. Once you start giving first aid, keep providing help until EMS personnel arrive.

LEGAL CONSIDERATIONS IN FIRST AID

Bystanders in an emergency are sometimes reluctant to help or give first aid to an ill or injured person. They may be afraid of being sued as a result of giving help, including first aid. Some legal concerns do exist. However, a caregiver of a child is legally obliged to help and, if necessary, give first aid. Fortunately, there are laws that protect First Aiders who help or give first aid to ill or injured persons.

The following obligations and protections apply to every caregiver. This includes parents, guardians, babysitters, and child care workers.

NOTE:

It is important to develop a policy that can be shared with parents and guardians. This would outline policies on providing first aid and/or medical attention.

NOTE:

If you are a child care worker:
- *you must provide first aid within your role as a child care worker*
- *you do not need the ill or injured child's permission to give help or first aid;*
- *however, if a parent or guardian is present, ask their permission.*

▶ Obligations

When a child is in your care, you are legally obliged to help and, if necessary, give first aid.

- You do not need the ill or injured child's permission to give help or first aid. Remember, there are different levels of help. Calling EMS/9-1-1 is providing first aid.

- When the child is not in your care, you are not obligated to help, but it is important that you treat others the way you would wish to be treated in the same situation.

- A parent or guardian cannot legally refuse to give consent if the situation is a life-threating one. If a parent or guardian will not let you help the child, have someone call EMS/9-1-1. Let them know the person has refused to let you help. The EMS personnel will deal with the situation.

▶ Protections

Most provinces and territories encourage bystanders to give first aid. The law provides that when you act reasonably and prudently under the conditions of an emergency, you cannot be held responsible for an aggravation of injury on the person. If you give first aid to an ill or injured person at the scene of an emergency, the law offers you some protection.

You must meet the following conditions:

- You must give assistance according to your level of training.
- You must not give assistance inside a hospital or other medical facility.
- Once you start to give first aid, you must continue until emergency medical service (EMS) personnel arrive.
- Your assistance must be voluntary. You must accept no reward for this assistance.
- You must not be guilty of gross negligence.
- You must act reasonably and prudently.

> **NOTE:**
>
> *In the province of Quebec, the Quebec civil code requires one to stop at the scene of an emergency and offer assistance, at minimum calling 9-1-1, or your local emergency number, and waiting for help to arrive.*

INFECTION

An **infection** is a disease caused by germs that invade your body.

You get an infection when:

1. there are germs in the environment around you;
2. the germs enter your body;
3. your immune system isn't strong enough to fight the germs; and
4. there are enough germs in your body to cause an infection.

If any one of these are missing, you won't get an infection.

▶ How Is an Infection Spread From One Person to Another?

There are four different ways that infections can be spread from one person to another:

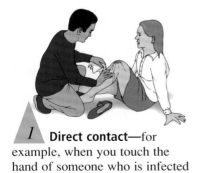

1 **Direct contact**—for example, when you touch the hand of someone who is infected

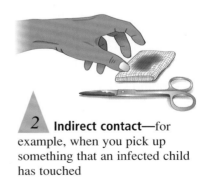

2 **Indirect contact**—for example, when you pick up something that an infected child has touched

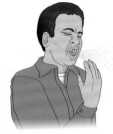

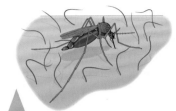

3 **Airborne transmission**—for example, when an infected child sneezes, sending germs into the air, and you breathe in those germs

4 **Vector transmission**—for example, when a mosquito bites an infected person and then bites you, passing on the germs

Some infections are spread through only one of these routes. Others may be spread through several possible routes.

There are some basic precautions you can take to stop infections, including diseases, from spreading.

▶ How to Prevent Diseases From Spreading

Figure 2.2 Clean toys and table tops daily.

- When you wash your hands, it is the rubbing and the soap that get rid of the germs, not the hot water.
- Toys must be cleaned daily in child care centres (Figure 2.2). To clean toys and equipment, use a solution of 3 mL of bleach to 200 mL of water. Label the bottle and make a fresh solution every day.
- In a child care setting, protect children from infectious diseases by:
    - ▶ insisting that staff who are sick NOT come into work;
    - ▶ encouraging parents to keep sick children at home;
    - ▶ having an isolation room for children who unexpectedly become ill;
    - ▶ wrapping sick children in a blanket or putting on an apron when you pick them up so that they don't come in direct contact with your clothes; and
    - ▶ washing your hands particularly well before and after you take care of a child who had diarrhea or is vomiting.

- In a child care setting, follow these guidelines when you're cleaning the bathroom:

    ▶ Clean and sanitize the bathroom sink, countertop, toilet, and floor with a bleach solution once a day and whenever it is obviously soiled.

    ▶ If you use the bathroom sink to clean potties, use a bleach solution to sanitize the sink afterwards.

- Wash bedding and equipment at least once a week. Wash them every day when children are sick.

> **NOTE:**
> *You must use personal protective equipment in the workplace. However, if you are helping a family member, it is your choice as to whether you use personal protective equipment.*

Direct and Indirect Contact

- Always be extremely careful when handling potentially contaminated objects.
- Avoid touching or being splashed by body fluids. Place an effective barrier, such as gloves, between you and the injured child's body fluids.
- Use a barrier device, such as a pocket mask, when doing CPR.
- Follow the handwashing techniques described in this chapter.

Airborne Transmission

- It's important to teach children the importance of covering their mouths when they cough or sneeze and of washing their hands afterwards.

Vector Transmission

- Wear protective clothing and use insect repellent when at risk of bites from insects.

Disposable Gloves

When you take off a pair of gloves, make sure that the outside of the glove doesn't touch your skin (Figure 2.3). Always wash your hands after you take off gloves.

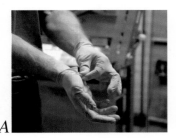 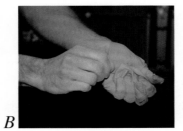 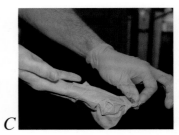

A B C

Figure 2.3 *A–C*: Safe glove removal.

Some people are allergic to latex. For some people, latex causes a mild skin rash. For others, it can cause a life-threatening reaction called *anaphylaxis*. When you're giving first aid, always check for MedicAlert® medical identification products that will tell you if the person has a serious illness or allergy.

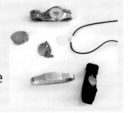

 Hand Washing to Avoid Spreading Germs

Hand washing is an important precaution wherever you are. It helps prevent spreading germs that can cause many infectious diseases.

When to Wash Your Hands

As a caregiver or First Aider, you should wash your hands before and after activities such as the following:

- Handling food and eating
- Diapering a child
- Going to the toilet or helping a child with toilet training
- Handling pets and/or cleaning animal cages
- Going on personal breaks
- Blowing or wiping noses
- Dealing with an open wound
- Attending to a sick child

Children should wash their hands before and after:

- Eating or handling food
- Water play
- Sand play
- Playing with play dough

Children should wash their hands after:

- Having a diaper changed
- Using the toilet
- Playing outdoors or in sand
- Playing with pets or animals
- Being touched by a child who may be ill

Hand Washing Procedures

Use the following guidelines for washing your hands:

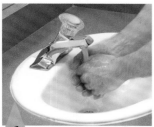

1 Always use warm running water and a mild soap. Use liquid soap if possible. You can use an antibacterial soap if you want to, but it isn't necessary.

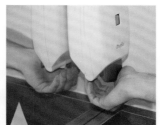

2 Wet your hands and apply a small amount of soap, about the size of a dime or a quarter.

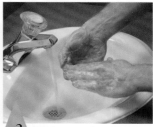

3 Rub your hands together vigorously until you see a soapy lather. Keep rubbing your hands for at least 15 seconds. Make sure you scrub between your fingers, under your fingernails, and around the backs and palms of your hands.

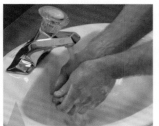

4 Rinse your hands under warm running water. Leave the water running while you dry your hands.

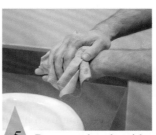

5 Dry your hands with a clean, disposable towel. Be careful not to touch the faucet handles or the towel holder with your clean hands.

7 Throw the used towel into a trash can that is lined with a plastic bag. Trash cans with lids that you can open with a foot pedal are best.

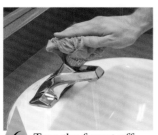

6 Turn the faucet off using the towel as a barrier between your hands and the faucet handle.

NOTE:

Child care centres, recreational centres, social organizations, schools, offices, and other workplaces are governed by public health and workplace health and safety guidelines and regulations. If you work in one of these environments, learn the specific local, provincial/territorial, or organizational laws and regulations that apply to your setting.

Diapering

A good diapering routine will greatly reduce the spread of germs that cause diarrhea. It will also leave children's skin clean and dry and make it less likely that they will develop diaper rash. You can also help reduce the spread of diarrhea by having infants and toddlers wear clothes over top of their diapers. Where you change a diaper is as important as how you change it.

Follow these steps when you change a diaper:

1 Check the diaper every hour and change it if it is soiled or wet.

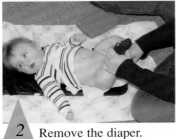

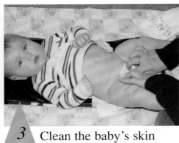

2 Remove the diaper.

3 Clean the baby's skin with warm water and then dry it well. Use soap only if the baby has had a bowel movement.

4 Use diaper cream only if the baby has a rash or the skin is red as cream can trap germs, urine, and stool on the skin. Creams are also very hard to wash off the skin, so spread the ointment thinly with a facial tissue. Take extra care cleaning and drying the skin with each diaper change. Powders can get in the air and the baby can inhale them, so use creams as opposed to talc, baby powder, or cornstarch.

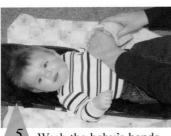

5 Wash the baby's hands and then move the baby to a safe place.

6 Wash your own hands. See page 11 for handwashing procedures.

How do you change a diaper in a sanitary way?

- Use disposable gloves and remove them before sanitizing the area.
- Set up your change table close to running water, away from the kitchen or eating area.
- Ensure that the change table is cleaned for at least 30 seconds with a bleach solution after each diapering.
- Dispose of dirty cloth diapers into a diaper pail with a snug-fitting lid. Diaper pails and garbage cans need to be put out of children's reach.
- Place disposable diapers into the garbage can immediately.
- Avoid washing soiled clothes. Place them in a sealed plastic bag to be picked up by the parent at the end of the day.

▶ Immunization as a Personal Precaution

Most people have been immunized against common childhood diseases, such as measles and mumps (Figure 2.4). Immunization introduces a substance into your body that builds up your resistance against the germs that cause a specific disease.

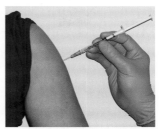

Figure 2.4 Immunization helps prevent illness and disease.

Children usually get immunizations because they are required for school or sports programs. However, not all adults have been immunized. Talk to your doctor or local community health nurse about your immunizations.

DENTAL HEALTH

- Encourage children to brush their teeth every day.
    - ▶ A good time to brush is right after lunch. Use a pea-sized amount of toothpaste that contains fluoride (Figure 2.5).
    - ▶ Rinse the toothbrush well. When you put it away, make sure it is not touching other toothbrushes.

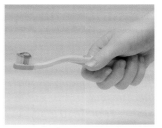

Figure 2.5 A pea-sized amount of toothpaste.

-
    - ▶ Replace the brush when the bristles become flattened.
    - ▶ Supervise young children when they are brushing.
- Children's and babies' teeth can decay if they nap with a bottle because their soft teeth are constantly exposed to liquid with sugar. This is called nursing bottle syndrome, and it can be caused by:
    - ▶ Cow's milk
    - ▶ Formula
    - ▶ Juice
    - ▶ Sweetened liquids

> **NOTE:**
>
> *Signs of decay include:*
> *• dull, white, or brown spots on the teeth.*

- When children are between the ages of one and two, encourage them to start drinking from a cup instead of from a bottle.
- Don't put honey, sugar, or syrup on soothers.
- Serve well-balanced meals. Too much sugary food is not healthy.

PREPARING FOR EMERGENCIES

By being prepared for emergencies, you can make sure that an ill or injured person gets help as soon as possible. First aid training gives you a plan of action for any emergency and gives you the confidence to act.

Make sure your family and co-workers know what to do in all types of emergencies. In addition, it is important to be familiar with any emergency guidelines that pertain to your jurisdiction.

Here are other important actions to take to prepare for an emergency in advance:

• Maintain up-to-date training in first aid and CPR.

• Post all emergency numbers near every telephone in your home and in your place of work.

• Draw up an emergency plan. Practise the plan with staff and children in a way that will not frighten the children.

• Keep a first aid kit in your home and your place of work.

• Make sure all emergency equipment is in good working order.

AFTER AN EMERGENCY

After dealing with an emergency it is often helpful to talk to somebody about the situation. If you are really bothered, contact someone who is trained in crisis intervention. You can contact your local crisis intervention line or look in the front of your phone book for information on whom to contact.

As a First Aider you can help others involved in the emergency by talking to them and providing comfort.

If emergencies happen in the workplace, fill out the proper forms or incident reports afterwards.

Debriefing after emergencies and reviewing injury reports regularly can help you identify and manage injuries more effectively.

PREPARING FOR DISASTERS

Disasters and personal emergencies can and do happen anywhere in Canada.

The key to being prepared is to identify what disasters could happen in your home, in a child care setting, or in another workplace or recreational facility.

NOTE:

The following are general guidelines. Child care centres and other workplaces will have to conform to laws and regulations that govern them for emergency and disaster preparedness.

- Talk with your family and co-workers about the dangers of fire, severe weather, and other disasters that could happen in your area. Discuss how you would respond to each type of disaster.

- Have parents pick one contact person (e.g., a friend or relative) nearby and one farther away for family members to call in case of disaster.

- Pick two meeting places: one near your home or child care centre to use in case of fire and one outside the neighbourhood to use in case you cannot return after a disaster.

- Keep vital records in a waterproof and fireproof container.

- Have emergency supply kits handy at home, at the child care centre or other workplace or recreational facility, and in your car.

NOTE:

For more information visit the Disaster Services page at www.redcross.ca.

AFTER A DISASTER

- Move people away from unsafe areas.

- Unless you need to call EMS/9-1-1, don't use the telephone.

- If you have been separated from your family, co-workers, or children under your care, register with the local Red Cross.

- If you have to evacuate, wear sturdy shoes and clothing that will keep you comfortable. Take your emergency supplies kit. Lock the building when you leave unless otherwise advised or in case of fire.

The Emergency Medical Services System

You're walking into the house with your two-month-old son still buckled in his baby car seat and you trip and fall, landing with your son still in your arms. You're unhurt from the fall, but the baby seat gets knocked pretty hard. You quickly check your son, who appears to be okay, but it's hard to tell as he starts screaming at the top of his lungs. A minute later, he suddenly stops crying and falls asleep. You try waking him up but can't. You run for the phone and call 9-1-1.

THE EMERGENCY MEDICAL SERVICES SYSTEM

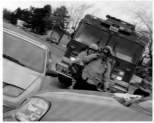

Figure 3.1 An EMS person in action.

The emergency medical services (EMS) system is a network of community resources and personnel organized to give emergency care in cases of injury or sudden illness. The system varies from community to community. In many areas, you can call 9-1-1, whereas other areas have a different local number. The level of training of EMS personnel may also vary, but the overall system and the principles of calling EMS are the same in every province and territory (Figure 3.1).

WHEN TO CALL EMERGENCY MEDICAL SERVICES (EMS)/9-1-1

As a general rule, call EMS/9-1-1 in cases of:

• Unconsciousness or an altered level of consciousness

• Difficulty breathing or no breathing

• Deadly bleeding

• Blood in the vomit, urine, or stool

• Seizure, severe headache, or slurred speech

• Injuries to the head, neck, or back

• Possible broken bones

Always call EMS/9-1-1 if the situation involves any of the following:

- Fire or explosion
- Live electrical wires
- Motor vehicle collision
- Swift-moving water
- Poisonous gas
- A situation where you cannot get to the person easily

WHEN TO CALL PARENTS OR GUARDIANS

- Fever
- Diarrhea
- Vomiting

> **NOTE:**
> *When in doubt, call EMS/9-1-1 and parents or guardians.*

- Any injury to the body (for a minor wound, such as a small cut, you would not call parents or guardians but would need to make them aware of it when they pick up their child)
- Child doesn't play or shows other abnormal behaviour
- Loss of or decrease in normal appetite

HOW TO CALL EMERGENCY MEDICAL SERVICES (EMS)/9-1-1

1. Make sure that emergency numbers are posted near every telephone in your home and at the child care centre, other place of work, or recreational facility (Figure 3.2). Many areas have a 9-1-1 number; others use a local number.

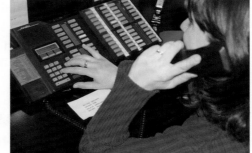

2. When you call EMS/9-1-1, this is what will happen in most communities:

Figure 3.2 Post emergency numbers by the phone.

- A dispatcher will answer. This dispatcher will be in a communication centre.
- You will supply details about the emergency. Most dispatchers will ask for the following information:
  - ▶ Specific location of the emergency
  - ▶ Telephone number from which the call is being made
  - ▶ Caller's name
  - ▶ How many people are involved

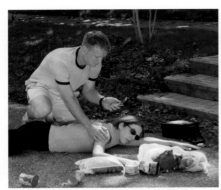
Figure 3.3 Do not hang up until the dispatcher tells you to do so.

▶ Condition of the child

▶ What is being done for the child

• A decision will then be made about how to respond. The decision may be to send police, ambulance personnel, firefighters, or a combination of personnel.

• It is very important that you do not hang up until the dispatcher tells you to do so (Figure 3.3).

• If the child is unresponsive or you feel immediate medical attention is necessary, shout for help. Then send someone to call EMS/9-1-1. If you are alone, you must make the call.

WHAT TO DO AFTER YOU HAVE CALLED EMS/9-1-1

• Call another caregiver or trusted neighbour to come and stay with any other children in your care.

• Call the ill or injured child's parents or guardians and ask them to meet you at the hospital. Tell them you will call again when you know the name and location of the hospital and that this may not be until you arrive.

• If you cannot go with the child in the ambulance, be sure to give the ambulance personnel the child's medical information and your phone number.

WHAT TO DO IF THE EMS/9-1-1 DISPATCHER TELLS YOU TO TAKE THE CHILD TO THE HOSPITAL

• Call another caregiver or trusted neighbour to come and stay with any other children in your care.

• Call the child's parents or guardians and ask them to meet you at the hospital.

• Ask someone else to drive you or call a taxi. (Do not drive alone.)

• As a last resort, call an ambulance to transport the child to the hospital.

• Take the child's medical information to the hospital.

Check, Call, Care

The last parent has just dropped off his son at the child care centre and you are starting the program for the day. Just then, a child screams from the other side of the room. She has fallen off a chair and landed on her head. There appears to be bleeding from a wound. You remember the Check, Call, Care steps from your first aid and CPR course. You go to help the injured girl.

PRIMARY SURVEY

 Check

Check the Scene

- Is the scene of the emergency safe?
- What happened?
- How many people are ill or injured?
- Can others help?

> **LOOK OUT FOR...**
> *Keep safe! Enter a scene only if it is safe to do so.*

Check the Child

The ill or injured child will be in one of the following states:

- Conscious: responsive; may be alert
- Confused: not responsive; not able to answer questions; seems disoriented
- Unresponsive: not awake

These states can be progressive; you can move from one to another or move within one of the states (e.g., when conscious you may be alert and then move to being not alert).

- If a child seems to be unresponsive and it is safe to do so, approach the child and ask, "Are you okay?" Use the child's name if you know it.
- Tap the child on the shoulder.
- If there is no response, EMS/9-1-1 must be contacted.

> **NOTE:**
> *Instead of tapping a baby on the shoulder, clap loudly and gently flick the bottom of the feet.*

▶ Call

- Shout for help. Have someone call EMS/9-1-1.
- If you are alone or no one else can call, you must make the call. If you are alone and the child or baby requires CPR, do 5 cycles (2 minutes) of CPR first, then call EMS/9-1-1.
- Ask someone for help.

▶ Care

Immediate Care

LOOK OUT FOR...
If there is a problem with the ABCs, it must be treated right away as it is a life-threatening emergency.

A: Airway

- Open the ill or injured child's airway using the head-tilt/chin-lift.

B: Breathing

- Check for normal breathing for no more than 10 seconds.

C: Circulation

- Look for deadly bleeding. Check from head to toe. Look for signs of shock.

SHOCK

Shock is oxygen starvation in the brain and other vital organs. This can be caused by blood loss, fluid loss, emotion, illness, or injury. Treating for shock may save an ill or injured child's life.

LOOK OUT FOR...
A child should be treated for shock before the signs appear. This is because children do not always show the early signs of shock.

▶ What to Look For

- Anxiety
- Confusion
- Cold, clammy skin
- Unconsciousness
- Skin that is paler than normal
- Weakness
- Nausea and vomiting

NOTE:
Shock can be caused by heavy bleeding, severe burns, pain, or fear. Shock can lead to death. Treat the cause, as well as the shock. It is extremely important to treat every child for shock.

What to Do

NOTE:

Follow the Check, Call, Care steps.

1 Shout for help. Have someone call EMS/9-1-1. If you are alone or no one else can call, you must make the call.

2 Care for the cause of the shock.

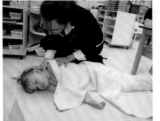

4 Monitor the ABCs.

5 Help the child get into a comfortable position.

3 Cover the ill or injured child lightly, or as needed, to maintain normal body temperature.

6 Comfort and reassure the child.

SECONDARY SURVEY

NOTE:

Only move on to a secondary survey if the ABCs are present.

If the child's ABCs are present, you need to find out what else may be wrong. To do this, you should do a secondary survey of the child to look for injuries that are non-life-threatening at this point in time. There are three parts to this:

1. Ask **questions**. Interview the child (if conscious) and other people at the scene to get more information.

2. Check **vital signs**. Look for level of consciousness, breathing, and skin colour.

   Skin that is paler than usual and lips that are bluish indicate problems with circulation.

3. Check the child for injuries from **head to toe**.

If you can, write down what you find during the secondary survey or have someone else write it down or help you remember. When EMS personnel arrive, give them the notes or tell them what you learned.

NOTE:

Always complete the secondary survey before treating any non-life-threatening injuries. If the child has minor bleeding, have them hold a clean cloth or gauze pad over the wound while you complete the survey.

▶ Ask Questions

- Interview the ill or injured child; simple questions are best.
  Here are some examples:
    - ▶ What happened?
    - ▶ How do you feel?
    - ▶ Where does it hurt?
    - ▶ Are you hungry? Are you thirsty?

Signs are signals of illness or injury that a First Aider can see, hear, or feel when checking the ill or injured child.

Symptoms are things the ill or injured child says that he or she feels.

▶ Check Vital Signs

- Level of Consciousness
    - ▶ *Is the ill or injured child awake or sleepy? confused? unresponsive?*
- Breathing
    - ▶ *Listen for sounds. Is the ill or injured child breathing quickly or slowly? Does it hurt her to breathe?*
- Skin
    - ▶ *Is the skin dry, wet, an unusual colour? What is the temperature?*

Feel the child's forehead with the back of your hand. In comparison to the environment she is in, does she seem too warm or too cool?

▶ Head-to-Toe Check: Hands Off

A head-to-toe check is done after the ABCs are okay and there are no life-threatening emergencies. Now you are looking for non-life-threatening injuries.

If the child is conscious and you are able to ask her questions, do a hands-off check.

If the child's level of consciousness changes or if any problems develop, *stop* whatever you are doing and give first aid *immediately*.

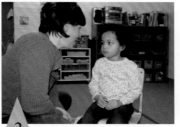

1 Start by telling the child what you are going to do and ask her to stay still.

2 Look at all areas of the body that are not covered by clothing for discoloration (bruises) or deformities (odd shapes).

A MedicAlert® medical identification product indicates that the child wearing it has a particular medical condition. These products include bracelets, necklaces, watch straps, wallet cards, and anklets.

3 Look at the appearance of the skin and check its temperature with the back of your hand. For privacy reasons, remove articles of clothing only if the clothing is hindering first aid.

4 Look for a MedicAlert® medical identification product. This tag may tell you what might be wrong, whom to call for help, and what care to give.

5 Ask the child to move each body part one at a time to see if anything hurts. If you suspect a head or spinal injury, do not have the child move any body parts.

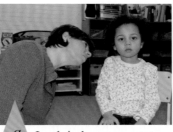

a Look in her ears, nose, and mouth for blood or fluids.

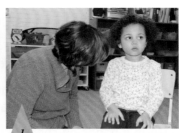

b If she has neck pain, do not move the neck. If there is no neck pain, ask her to slowly move her head from side to side.

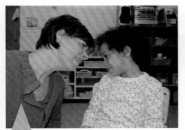

c Ask the child to shrug her shoulders. Ask if there is any pain or discomfort.

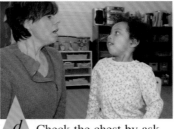

d Check the chest by asking the child to take a deep breath and then blow the air out.

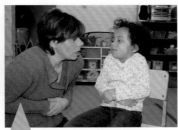

e Check the abdomen by asking the child to push her stomach out and then pull it in.

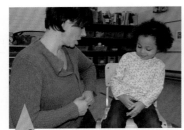

f Check the hips by asking the child to move them slightly.

Ask the child to wiggle her toes if there is no pain in the hips.

- Have her move her ankles if there is no pain in the toes.
- Ask her to move her knees by bending if there is no pain in the ankles.

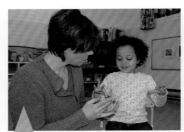

g Check the hands by asking the child to wiggle her fingers.

- If there is no pain in the fingers, have her move her wrists.
- If there is no pain in the wrists, have her move her elbows.

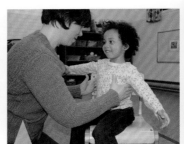

6 If the child doesn't complain of any pain and doesn't have any tender areas or signs of injury, ask the child to rest for a few minutes in a comfortable position. Check the vital signs and monitor the ABCs. If you see no problem, help the child stand up slowly when she is ready.

7 If the child has pain or dizziness or cannot move a body part or if you found any injuries, provide first aid and, if needed, call EMS/9-1-1.

▶ Head-to-Toe Check: Hands-On

This check is mainly for an unconscious child who cannot tell you what is wrong. If the child is conscious, you may need to do a hands-on check at the site of the injury.

Perform a hands-on check only if you can be sure that the airway will not be compromised.

Remember to wear your gloves when performing the hands-on check.

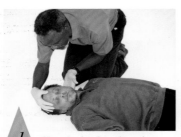

1 Check the head and neck; look and feel for any abnormalities, such as bumps, soft spots, or bleeding.

- Soft spots may mean a fracture of the skull, so do not push on these spots.

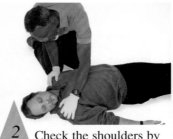

2 Check the shoulders by looking and feeling for any bumps or bone deformities.

> **NOTE:**
>
> *As you do this check, keep watching the person's level of consciousness, breathing, and skin (vital signs). If any problems develop, stop whatever you are doing and give first aid immediately.*

LOOK OUT FOR...

Be careful not to reach underneath someone as there could be objects such as glass, which could cause injury. Look around and under the body for any signs of blood or fluids.

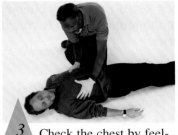

3 Check the chest by feeling the ribs for deformity.

- When the person breathes, both sides of the rib cage should expand at the same time. If any part of the ribs move differently from the rest when the person breathes, call EMS/9-1-1.

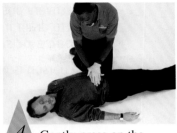

4 Gently press on the abdomen to see if it is hard.

- The abdomen should feel soft to the touch.
- If the abdomen is painful or hard to the touch, you may have to move clothing and check for bruising.
- Do not poke or push on a hard, painful, or bruised abdomen.

5 To check the hips, put your hands on both sides of the pelvis and push down on the hip bones and then in on the sides.

- The hip bones should move together.
- If the person shows any signs of discomfort, refrain from pushing or pulling.

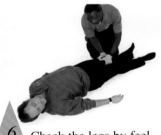

6 Check the legs by feeling for any deformity in the bones or for swelling.

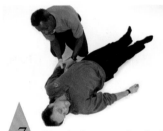

7 Check the arms by feeling for any deformity in the bones or for swelling.

CONTINUAL CARE

After your secondary survey it is important to keep the child comfortable and monitor the ABCs continually until EMS personnel arrive.

▶ Recovery Position

Once you've checked the ABCs, you should move an unconscious child into the *recovery position* if:

1. The airway is open;
2. The child is breathing;
3. There is no serious bleeding; and
4. You don't suspect a neck or back injury.

The recovery position keeps the airway open and allows any blood or vomit to drain from the mouth, which is why it's also called the **drainage position**.

If the person is on her back:

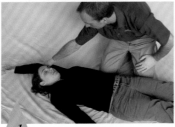

1 Raise the arm closest to you.

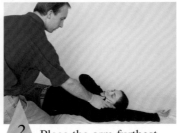

2 Place the arm furthest from you across the person's chest with the palm against the cheek.

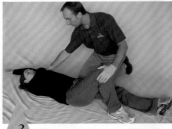

3 Raise the knee of the leg furthest away from you.

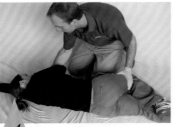

4 Support the head and neck with one hand as you pull the person towards you with your other hand on the raised leg close to the knee.

5 Position the person on his or her side with knee out in front and hip at right angle to prevent the person from rolling onto his or her face.

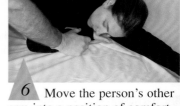

6 Move the person's other arm into a position of comfort in front of the body.

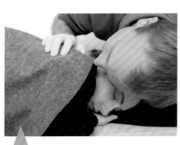

7 With the person's head resting on the extended arm, tilt the head and open the mouth to clear the way for drainage.

The person should now be positioned on his or her side, and you can remove your hand. Check the airway to ensure that it is clear. Treat for shock.

Airway Emergencies

It is a lovely summer day, and you are sitting in your sister's backyard, taking care of her children. She has gone shopping and said she would be back in two hours. Suddenly, her two-year-old son starts choking. He was playing on the lawn not far from your chair. Could he have picked up something and put it in his mouth? You remember your first aid training and shout for help. Then you send your sister's five-year-old son to call EMS/9-1-1.

The airway is the passage that connects the nose and mouth with the lungs. If anything blocks the airway, the person chokes and cannot get enough oxygen. This is a life-threatening emergency, and you must give first aid to remove whatever is blocking the airway.

CHOKING

NOTE:

Severe choking happens when the airway is completely blocked.

Choking happens when a foreign object blocks the airway. The object may get stuck at any point in the airway from the throat to the lungs. Choking can affect adults, children, and babies.

There are other ways that the airway can get blocked. For example, an allergic reaction can make the airway swell up or the tongue can block the airway when a person is unconscious.

NOTE:

Coughing is an indicator of mild choking. Encourage the child to keep coughing.

 ### Causes of Choking

The following are causes of choking in children:

- Laughing or talking while eating
- Improperly chewing food

Children may be especially prone to choke because they:

- Eat food cut into pieces that are too big

- Put objects in their mouths (e.g., small toys or coins)
- Run or walk while eating or chewing gum or candy

▶ Prevention

- When babies start eating solid food, start with puréed food, as opposed to pieces of food. Then give them mashed food. Eventually, small pieces can be offered.
- Always supervise babies when they are eating.
- When babies are teething, you may want to give food for comfort. Offer a soother or toast instead of hard vegetables, which may get stuck in the throat.
- Use unbreakable cups and dishes and a spoon, not a fork.
- Teach children in your care to eat calmly and chew properly.
- Teach children in your care not to speak with a mouthful of food.
- Encourage children to sit while eating.
- Be sure that children's booster seats or hook-on chairs are safe. They should have a harness. They should also be secured to a regular chair.

> **NOTE:**
> *The most common causes in children are:*
> - *Balloons*
> - *Small objects*
> - *Foods (e.g., hot dogs, hard candies, nuts, and grapes)*
> - *Liquids can cause choking too, especially in babies.*

FOODS THAT CAUSE CHOKING AND PREVENTATIVE SAFETY MEASURES[1]

The following foods are known to have caused choking in children. Safety measures you can take are shown in the right-hand column.

Food	Safety Measure
Hot dogs	Avoid
Other meats	Grind
Nuts	Avoid
Popcorn	Avoid
Hard candy	Avoid
Fruit with seeds	Remove seeds
Fruits and vegetables	Shred
Grapes	Avoid
Peanut butter	Avoid

[1]Alberta Safe and Secure Manual.

▶ **What to Look For**

- Distressed facial expression
- Mouth open
- Not breathing
- Not coughing
- Making a high-pitched noise
- Clutching the throat
- Change in face colour (bluish or paler than normal)

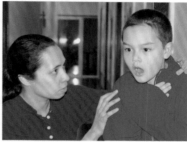

Figure 5.1 Encourage the child to cough up the foreign object.

If the child can breathe, speak, or cough forcefully, encourage him to cough up the foreign object (Figure 5.1).

Stay with the child and monitor closely. Hitting the child on the back could cause the object to become lodged even further in the throat.

 ## **What to Do**

Conscious Child Choking

If the child is unable to speak or breathe or has wheezing breathing:

NOTE:

To determine if choking is mild or severe: Ask, "Are you choking?" If the child can speak, cough, or breathe, it is mild choking. Encourage him to continue coughing and do not interfere. The obstruction might clear itself.

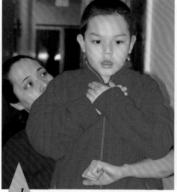

1 Stand (or kneel for a small child) behind the child and wrap both arms around the abdomen.

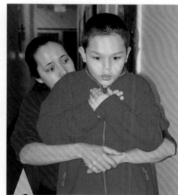

2 Make a fist and place it just above the belly button and lower rib cage.

- Place your other hand over the fist and pull sharply in and up.
- Continue until the object comes out or the child becomes unconscious.

If the child becomes unconscious, shout for help. Have someone call EMS/9-1-1. If you are alone or if no one else can call, you must make the call. Then follow the steps for unconscious choking.

> **NOTE:**
> *A child is between the ages of 1 and 8.*

Unconscious Child Choking

Check

- Check the scene for danger.
- If safe to do so, check the child.

Call

If the child is unresponsive, have someone call EMS/9-1-1 and get an automated external defibrillator (AED) if one is available.

Care

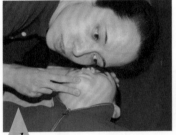

1 Open the airway using the head-tilt/chin-lift and check for normal breathing for 5 to 10 seconds:

- Look, listen, and feel.

2 If you do not hear normal breathing, give two rescue breaths:

- Pinch the nose.
- Take a normal breath.
- Cover the person's mouth with your mouth.
- Give two breaths; each breath should last one second, with just enough volume to make the chest rise.

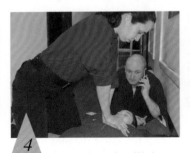

3 If the child's chest does not rise after the first breath, perform the head-tilt/chin-lift again and attempt to give a breath.

4 If your breath still does not go in, start CPR:

- Place the heel of one hand in the middle of the child's chest. Place the other hand on top.
- Do 30 compressions: "Push hard, push fast."
- Allow the chest to recoil.

> **NOTE:**
> *Remember your gloves and other barrier devices.*

"Push hard, push fast"

Compression depths:

Older Child – 4 to 5 cm (1.5 to 2 in)

Child/Baby – 1/3 to 1/2 the depth of the chest

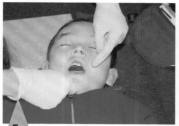

5a After each cycle of compressions, look in the mouth.

- Grasp both the tongue and lower jaw between your thumb and fingers and lift the jaw.
- If you do not see an object, try to give a breath, if breath does not go in, go to Step 4.
- If you see an object, remove it and go to Step 6.

NOTE:
If your breath does not go in, go back to compressions.

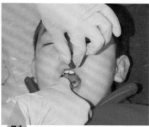

5b Slide your finger down the inside of the cheek to the base of the tongue and try to sweep the object out.

NOTE:
If there is any change in the child's condition during CPR, stop and check the child's ABCs.

6 Give a breath. If your first breath goes in, give a second breath.

7 When both breaths go in and there is no obvious response to your two breaths, start the CPR sequence of 30 compressions and 2 breaths.

Conscious Baby Choking

Check

- Check the scene for danger.
- If safe to do so, check the baby.

Call

- Shout for help

Care

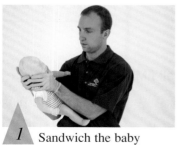

1 Sandwich the baby between your forearms, supporting the head.

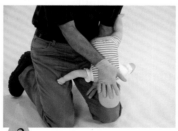

2 Turn the baby face down, with the head lower than the body.

NOTE:
If a baby is coughing or gagging the choking is mild. Do not interfere. If the baby is making high-pitched noises, wheezing, can no longer make a sound or becomes too weak to cough:
- *Send someone to call EMS/9-1-1.*

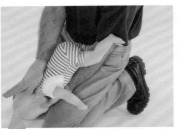

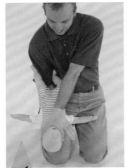

3 Lower your forearm onto your thigh. With the heel of your hand, deliver five back blows between the shoulder blades.

4 While still supporting the head, turn the baby face up, with your arm supported on your thigh.

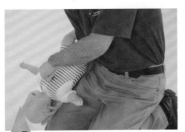

5 Place two fingers on the centre chest just below the nipple line and "push hard, push fast" $\frac{1}{3}$ to $\frac{1}{2}$ the depth of the chest five times.

• Repeat the back blows and chest thrusts until the object is coughed up; the baby starts to cry, breathe, or cough; or the baby becomes unconscious.

If the baby becomes unconscious, follow the steps for unconscious choking.

Unconscious Baby Choking

Check

• Check the scene for danger.

• If safe to do so, check the baby.

Call

If the baby is unresponsive, send someone to call EMS/9-1-1.

Care

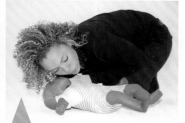

1 Open the airway using the head-tilt/chin-lift and check for normal breathing for 5 to 10 seconds:

- Look, listen, and feel.

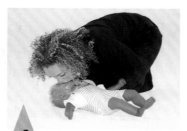

2 If you do not hear normal breathing, give two gentle breaths:

- Take a normal breath.
- Seal your lips tightly over the baby's mouth and nose.
- Give two breaths; each breath should last one second, with enough volume to make the chest rise.

3 If the baby's chest does not rise after the first breath, perform the head-tilt/chin-lift again and attempt to give a breath.

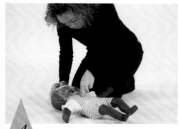

4 If your breath still does not go in, start CPR:

- Place two fingers on the middle of the chest, just below the nipple line.
- Do 30 compressions. "Push hard, push fast."

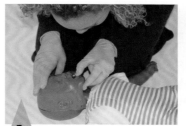

5a After each cycle of compressions, look in the mouth.

- Grasp both the tongue and lower jaw between your thumb and fingers and lift.
- If you do not see an object, try to give a breath, if breath does not go in, go to Step 4.
- If you see an object, remove it and go to Step 6.

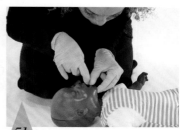

5b Slide your finger down the inside of the cheek to the base of the tongue and try to sweep the object out.

> **NOTE:**
>
> *If your breath does not go in, go back to compressions.*

6 Give a breath. If the first breath goes in, give a second breath.

7 When both breaths go in and if there is no obvious response to your 2 breaths, start the CPR sequence of 30 compressions and 2 breaths.

> **NOTE:**
>
> *If there is any change in the baby's condition during CPR, stop and check the baby's ABCs.*

Breathing and Circulation Emergencies

After lunch, the children at the child care centre head outside to play. It's a warm fall day, but not too hot. One of the boys takes a soccer ball away from a younger girl who suffers from asthma. The young girl chases after the boy but stops beside a tree and hangs onto the trunk. She starts wheezing and gasping for air. You rush over to her and take her inside.

BREATHING EMERGENCIES

A person having difficulty breathing is in **respiratory distress**. A person who can't breathe at all is in **respiratory arrest**. Both respiratory distress and respiratory arrest are **breathing emergencies**.

HYPERVENTILATION

NOTE:

Children's hearts stop due to breathing emergencies, so it is important to treat them as soon as possible.

Hyperventilation occurs when breathing is faster than normal. This upsets the body's balance of oxygen and carbon dioxide.

 Causes

Hyperventilation is often triggered by an upsetting situation but can also be caused by injury.

 What to Look For

- Rapid, shallow breathing
- Dizziness
- Panic
- Anxiety

LOOK OUT FOR...

If there are signs and symptoms of an injury, the hyperventilation doesn't stop after a few minutes, or the child becomes unconscious, shout for help. Have someone call EMS/ 9-1-1. If alone, you must make the call.

 What to Do

1. Comfort the child. Encourage her to take long, slow breaths and to hold her breath before breathing out slowly.

NOTE:

Follow the Check, Call, Care steps.

2. Treat any underlying injuries

3. If the child faints, follow the care for fainting. (See Chapter 11.)

ASTHMA ATTACK

In an *asthma attack*, the air passages become narrower and breathing is difficult. Asthma is more common in children and young adults than in adults. It is usually controlled with medication. Asthma attacks can come on very quickly.

 Causes

- Excessive physical activity
- Stress
- Allergic reactions

 Prevention

Asthma attacks can be prevented or lessened if sufferers take their prescribed medications. It is also important for sufferers to avoid the following:

- Cold and flu
- Both extreme dryness and extreme humidity
- Emotional stress
- Temperature changes
- Cigarette smoke and other "trigger" substances

 What to Look For

- Coughing
- Difficulty breathing or speaking when exhaling
- Anxiety or restlessness
- Pale or bluish skin, especially around the lips and fingernails

 What to Do

As soon as you notice a child having an asthma attack:

1. Take the child to a quiet, well-ventilated area.
2. Seat her in a comfortable position.
3. Encourage or help the child to take her prescribed medication.
4. Comfort and reassure the child.
5. If the child is thirsty, offer sips of clear fluids.
6. Have the child sit near a cool mist vaporizer if one is available.
7. Be sure the child is warmly covered. It is important for her not to be chilled.

> **NOTE:**
>
> *Follow the Check, Call, Care steps.*

Call EMS/9-1-1 if:

- the child does not have a history of asthma;
- the attack is not helped by the child's prescribed medication; or
- the child cannot complete a sentence without gasping for air.

How to Help Someone Use an Inhaler (Puffer) With a Spacer[1]

1. Make sure that you have the inhaler that has been prescribed for that child. Ensure it is within the expiry date.

2. Shake the inhaler three or four times.

3. Remove the cap from the inhaler. If the child uses a spacer and it has a cap, remove it.

4. If the child uses a spacer, put the inhaler into the spacer.

5. Have the child breathe out, away from the inhaler and spacer.

> **NOTE:**
> *Most spacers for children come in the form of a mask.*

6. Bring the spacer or inhaler to the child's mouth, put the mouthpiece between her teeth, and tell her to close her lips around it.

7. Tell the child to press the top of the inhaler once. If she can't do it herself, you may do it for her.

8. Tell the child to take one slow, full breath, hold it for about 10 seconds, and then breathe out.

ALLERGIC REACTIONS

An *allergic reaction* is an exaggerated reaction of the body to a substance.

▶ Causes

Allergic reactions can be caused by food, dust, mould, or dander from pets, among other substances.

[1] Adapted from www.lung.ca

▶ **Prevention**

The following applies to caregivers other than parents or guardians (e.g., babysitters or child care workers). However, parents and guardians are involved in this prevention, too.

- Talk to the parents or guardians before you begin caring for the child.
- Ask the parents or guardians the following questions before the child comes into your care:
    - ▶ What is your child allergic to?
    - ▶ What signs will tell me that your child is having an allergic reaction?
    - ▶ What do you do if your child has a reaction?
    - ▶ Has the doctor prescribed any allergy medication? For instance, should you give us your child's epinephrine auto-injector?
- Make a list of the allergies of each child under your care. Keep it in a location where you can refer to it easily.
- Read all the ingredients on all food package labels and when cooking. Any foods containing ingredients to which the child is allergic should not be given.
- Before serving a new food, ensure that the parents or guardians have given it to the child at home and that there has been no allergic reaction (e.g., eggs, shellfish, milk, and wheat).
- If a child has to eat special foods, the parents or guardians should provide them.
- Post all food allergies in cooking and food service areas for easy reference.
- Avoid other allergy triggers, such as dust, pollen, fur, wasp or bee stings, and latex.

▶ **What to Look For**

- Generalized itching
- Blotches on the skin (Figure 6.1)
- Breathing difficulty
- Raised reddish swelling
- Nausea or vomiting
- Abdominal cramps
- Shock
- Tightness of the throat

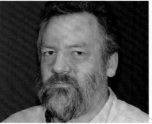

Figure 6.1 Rash, itching, or hives are a sign of an allergic reaction.

What to Do

<table>
<tr><td>**NOTE:**</td></tr>
</table>

- See What to Do under Anaphylaxis (Severe Allergic Reaction), below.

Follow the Check, Call, Care steps.

ANAPHYLAXIS (SEVERE ALLERGIC REACTION)

Anaphylaxis is a severe allergic reaction. The air passages swell, making breathing difficult. This could lead to respiratory arrest.

 ### Causes

Anaphylaxis may be caused by a severe reaction to an insect sting, food, or medicine.

 ### What to Look For

- Weakness
- Pale skin colour
- Difficulty breathing, wheezing
- Puffiness or swelling, especially near the eyes or throat
- Itchy skin (sometimes a rash will develop)
- In the case of a very severe reaction, the child may lose consciousness.

 ### What to Do

NOTE:

Follow the Check, Call, Care steps.

- If it is a severe allergic reaction, shout for help. Have someone call EMS/9-1-1. If alone, you must make the call.
- If the child has an epinephrine auto-injector, have the child use it immediately.
- Look for MedicAlert® medical identification products.
- Treat for shock. (See "What to Do" for shock in Chapter 4.)
- Apply a cold compress to the area (if the reaction is to a wasp or bee sting).
- If the child stops breathing, start cardiopulmonary resuscitation (CPR). (See Chapter 7.)

How to Use an Epinephrine Auto-injector

1. Before assisting with any medications, ensure that the Five Rights have been checked:

✔ Right person   ✔ Right drug

✔ Right dose   ✔ Right route

✔ Right time

2. Remove the grey safety cap.

3. Place the black tip against the child's outer thigh and with a quick motion push the auto-injector firmly against her thigh. You should hear a click.

4. Hold for 10 seconds.

5. Remove the epinephrine auto-injector.

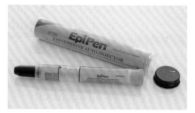

Figure 6.2 An epinephrine auto-injector.

Ensure that the used epinephrine auto-injector (Figure 6.2) goes to the hospital with the child.

▶ Comparison Chart for Epiglottitis and Croup

Both epiglottitis and croup affect the throat.

Table 6.1 *The Differences Between Epiglottitis and Croup*

	Epiglottitis	Croup
What is it?	Inflammation and swelling of the epiglottis. Not common among young children. When it strikes, it is life threatening.	Inflammation of the throat and vocal cords
Cause	Bacterial infection	Viral infection
Ages most likely to be affected	3 to 7 years old	6 months to 5 years old 5 years and older it is called laryngitis
Onset	Comes on suddenly, from 6 to 24 hours after infection	Develops more gradually, from 24 to 72 hours after infection
Child's appearance	Looks very ill and anxious	Looks only mildly or moderately ill
Drooling	Frequent; child has trouble swallowing saliva	No drooling
Hoarseness	Not usually	Very marked hoarseness
Coughing	Rare	Frequent, harsh "crowing" cough
What to do	Call EMS/9-1-1 immediately. If the child stops breathing, start CPR. (See Chapter 7.) Report the child's condition to the parents or guardians and/or doctor. **Do not inspect the mouth and/or throat.**	Have the child stay near a cool mist vaporizer. Report the child's condition to the parents or guardians and/or doctor. Doctors often recommend opening a window (if cool outside). They may also suggest stepping outside with a blanket wrapped around the child until the coughing ceases. A cold mist from a shower is also helpful.

RESPIRATORY ARREST

A person who stops breathing is in *respiratory arrest*. Without prompt first aid, respiratory distress can lead to respiratory arrest.

▶ Causes

- Strangulation
- Suffocation
- Drowning
- Poisoning
- Electrocution
- Severe allergy
- Airway obstruction
- Injury to head, chest, or lungs
- Respiratory conditions (such as asthma)

NOTE:

Follow the Check, Call, Care steps.

▶ What to Look For

- Child is unconscious
- Absence of normal breathing
- Bluish coloured lips and a face that is paler than normal

 ## What to Do

- Have someone call EMS/9-1-1. If you are alone, you must make the call.
- If the child stops breathing, start cardiopulmonary resuscitation (CPR). (See Chapter 7.)

▶ Prevention of Strangulation

- Ensure that hoods and scarves fit properly. They must be snugly tied and tucked. Otherwise, use neck warmers.
- Use clothing that does not have drawstrings as it may get caught in playground equipment.
- Remove strings from drapes and blinds.
- Use pacifier clips as opposed to cords.
- Discourage play with belts and ropes.
- Be careful with dress-up clothes and costumes.

▶ Prevention of Suffocation

- Keep all plastic bags and other plastic coverings out of the reach of children.
- Keep children away from plastic sheets (even those on mattresses) and balloons.
- Keep babies away from pillows.
- Lock or remove doors on unused appliances.
- Supervise babies nursing on a bottle.

- Children should not be placed on waterbeds.
- Remove lids from toy boxes.

▶ Prevention of Drowning

- Pay constant attention to babies or children when they are in or near water.
- Turn wading pools upside down when not in use.
- Fence private pools and have locking gates.
- Empty buckets of water immediately after use.
- Have a non-slip mat in the bathtub.
- Keep toilet lids down and keep the bathroom door closed.

CIRCULATION EMERGENCIES

All the children are napping, and it is time to awaken them. You notice that one of the babies is bluish in colour and not moving. You rush to the baby and begin CPR.

CARDIAC ARREST

Cardiac arrest happens when the heartbeat stops suddenly. In children, this is most often due to respiratory arrest.

▶ Causes

- Shaken Baby syndrome (SBS). (See Chapter 8.)
- Sudden Infant Death Syndrome (SIDS). This is also known as crib death.
- Electrical shock (If there are burns involved, see Chapter 10.)
- Respiratory arrest (See above.)
- Choking (See Chapter 5.)

▶ Prevention

- Use electrical wall protection plugs.
- Remove all electrical hazards when bathing children.
- Keep electrical cords away from children.

- Never shake a baby.
- Keep choking hazards away from children and babies.
- Teach children not to put items in their mouths that could make them choke.

 What to Look For

- Unresponsiveness
- Absence of normal breathing

NOTE:
Follow the Check, Call, Care steps.

 What to Do

1. Have someone call EMS/9-1-1. If you are alone, you must make the call.
2. Start CPR. (See Chapter 7.)

SUDDEN INFANT DEATH SYNDROME (SIDS)

SIDS, also known as crib death, is the unexpected death of an apparently healthy baby under one year of age.

Causes

- Usually occurs while the child is sleeping
- Remains unexplained even after a full investigation

Prevention

Nobody knows how to prevent SIDS.

To lessen the risk:

- Put a baby on her back to sleep.
- Make sure no one smokes around babies.
- Do not put too many clothes or covers on babies.
- Breastfeeding may give some protection against SIDS.

DEADLY BLEEDING

Deadly bleeding leads to large amounts of blood loss, either outside or within the body.

Causes

Deadly bleeding (Figure 6.3) can be caused by a sharp object, a severe fall, crushing pressure, or a sports injury.

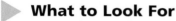 **Prevention**

- Keep all sharp objects, such as knives, in a safe place.
- Wear appropriate sports equipment.
- Prevent falls. (See Chapter 8.)

Figure 6.3 Deadly bleeding.

External Deadly Bleeding

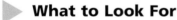 **What to Look For**

- Large amounts of blood loss.
- The child shows signs of shock.

NOTE:
Follow the Check, Call, Care steps.

 What to Do

- Have someone call EMS/9-1-1. If you are alone, you must make the call.
1. Put pressure directly on the wound.
2. Treat for shock. (See Chapter 4.)
3. If there are amputated body parts, send them with the child to the hospital.

NOTE:
Watch for bones or other objects sticking out of the wound.

Internal Deadly Bleeding

What to Look For

Internal bleeding is more difficult to recognize than external bleeding. It is not easy to look for signs and symptoms because they are inside. This means they are less obvious. They may also take time to appear.

- Bruising in the injured area
- Skin is tender, swollen, or hard
- Shock
- Severe thirst
- Pain
- Blood in saliva or vomit

What to Do

- Shout for help. Have someone call EMS/9-1-1. If you are alone, you must make the call.

NOTE:
Follow the Check, Call, Care steps.

1. Monitor the ABCs (airway, breathing, circulation) until EMS personnel arrive.
2. Help the ill or injured child rest in the most comfortable position possible.

First Aid for Respiratory and Cardiac Arrest

Your next-door neighbour bangs on the door. When you answer the door, you find her in a panic. Her five-year-old son had been playing in the backyard on the swing-set ladder when he slipped and fell. During his fall, his scarf caught on a bar and caused the scarf to tighten around his neck. She was able to get him safely down from the ladder and loosen the scarf, but he wasn't breathing. You rush over to help.

When a child or baby experiences a breathing emergency, such as an asthma attack or severe allergic reaction, breathing may stop. This is called **respiratory arrest**. All our body systems are related; once breathing stops, the heart will soon stop, which is called **cardiac arrest**.

Although children and babies don't suffer cardiovascular disease like adults do, they may experience cardiac arrest either when breathing stops or under certain emergencies, such as electric shock. Both respiratory arrest and cardiac arrest are life-threatening and need to be treated immediately.

CHILD CPR

 What to Do

Check

- Check the scene for danger.
- If safe to do so, check the child.

> **NOTE:**
>
> An older child is a child over the age of 8. For First Aid purposes, this is considered to be an adult.

Call

> **NOTE:**
>
> *If you are alone, you must make the call.*

If the child is unresponsive, shout for help. Have someone call EMS/9-1-1 and get an AED if one is available.

If you are alone with a child, do 5 cycles (two minutes) of CPR first, then call EMS/9-1-1 and return to care for the child. If you are alone with an older child (or adult), call right away.

Care

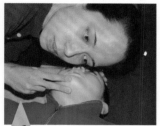

1 Open the airway using the head-tilt/chin-lift and check for breathing for 5 to 10 seconds:

- Look, listen, and feel.

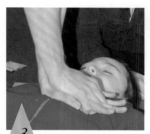

> **NOTE:**
> *If the child is face down, roll him over to assess breathing.*

3 If both breaths go in, start CPR:
- Place the heel of one hand in the middle of the child's chest. Place the other hand on top.
- Do 30 compressions: "Push hard, push fast."
- Allow the chest to recoil.
- Repeat cycles of compressions and breaths.

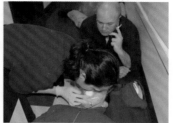

2 If you do not hear normal breathing, give two rescue breaths:

- Pinch the nose.
- Take a normal breath.
- Cover the child's mouth with your mouth.
- Give two breaths. Each breath should last one second, with enough volume to make the chest rise.

4 Continue CPR until:

- An AED arrives.
- More advanced care takes over.
- The scene becomes unsafe.
- You become physically unable to continue.

> **"Push hard, push fast"**
> Compression depths:
> Older Child – 4 to 5 cm (1.5 to 2 in)
> Child/Baby – 1/3 to 1/2 the depth of the chest

When the AED arrives:

1. Open and turn on the AED.
2. Remove any clothing or objects, including jewellery, that may come in contact with the pads.
3. Ensure that the chest is dry so the pads can stick.
4. Follow the diagrams on the pads to place them on the child. Use the appropriate pads for a child.
5. Follow the automated prompts of the AED.
6. When the AED prompts you to give a shock, stand clear and say, "I'm clear, you're clear, everybody's clear."

A child is between the ages of 1 and 8. For a child, use child pads. If no child pads are available, use adult pads. Follow the directions for pad placement. If there is less than 2.5 cm (1 in) between the pads when on the chest, place one on the front of the chest and one on the back.

▶ Public Access Defibrillation (PAD)

Public access defibrillation (PAD) is a movement to make AEDs readily available in many public areas, such as arenas or shopping centres. The advantage of AEDs is that it doesn't take much training to use them. With a little training and with voice prompts from the machine, users can successfully defibrillate someone in cardiac arrest. Contact your local city or municipality to find out more about the PAD program.

BABY CPR

 What to Do

Check

- Check the scene for danger.
- If safe to do so, check the baby.

Call

If the baby is unresponsive, shout for help. Have someone call EMS/9-1-1. If alone, you must make the call.

If you are alone with a baby, do 5 cycles (two minutes) of CPR first, then take the baby with you (as long as you don't suspect a head or spine injury) to call EMS/9-1-1.

Care

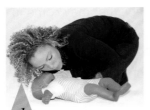

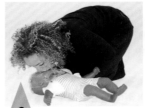

| NOTE: |
| *Do not tilt the head back too far.* |

 1 Open the airway using the head-tilt/chin-lift and check for normal breathing for 5 to 10 seconds:

- Look, listen, and feel.

2 If you do not hear normal breathing, give two gentle breaths:

- Take a normal breath.
- Seal your lips tightly over the baby's mouth and nose.
- Give two gentle breaths. Each breath should last one second, with just enough volume to make the chest rise.

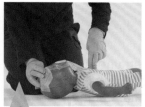

3 If both breaths go in, start CPR.

- Keep the airway open by using your hand to maintain a head-tilt.
- Place two fingers on the middle of the chest, just below the nipple line.
- Do 30 compressions: "Push hard, push fast."
- Allow the chest to recoil.
- Repeat cycles of compressions and breaths.

4 Continue CPR until:

- More advanced care takes over.
- The scene becomes unsafe.
- You become physically unable to continue.

IF YOU DISCOVER A BABY OR CHILD WHEN YOU ARE ALONE

 What to Do

Check

- Check the scene for danger.
- If safe to do so, check the child or baby.

Care

If the child or baby is unresponsive and you are alone, begin ABCs.

For a child (under the age of 8) or a baby, if there is no breathing, do 5 cycles (two minutes) of CPR and then put the child in the recovery position or take the baby with you to call EMS/9-1-1. Once the call has been made return to providing first aid.

You can always try shouting "Help" because someone may hear you. Remember to stay calm. If you are taking the baby with you, hold the baby securely and walk.

SPECIAL CONSIDERATIONS

 ### Air in the Stomach

Air in the stomach can make someone vomit. When an unconscious child vomits, the stomach contents may get into the lungs, a condition called *aspiration*. Aspiration makes giving rescue breaths more difficult, and it can be fatal.

 ### Vomiting

In some situations a child may vomit while you are giving CPR.

If this happens:

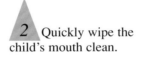

1 Turn the child's head and body together as one unit onto his side, facing you.

2 Quickly wipe the child's mouth clean.

3 Reposition the child on his back and continue with CPR.

 ### Mouth-to-Nose Breathing

Sometimes you cannot seal your mouth well over the child's mouth to give rescue breaths because:

• The child's jaw or mouth is injured or shut too tightly to open.

• Your mouth is too small to cover the child's mouth.

If this happens, breathe into the child's nose. Block his mouth to stop air from escaping.

Head and Spine Injuries

You've just put the children to bed, and you're settling into reading the newspaper when you hear a thump. It came from the direction of the bedroom your 10-year-old daughter shares with her 8-year-old sister. You run down the hall, turn on the bedroom lights, and find your eldest daughter wedged between the dresser and the bed. She's fallen from the top bunk and hit her head on the sharp corner of the dresser.

HEAD AND SPINE INJURIES

Head and spine injuries can be fatal. People who survive them can have physical and mental difficulties, including paralysis, speech problems, memory problems, and behavioural disorders. Many people with these injuries are permanently disabled.

 Causes

The causes of head and spine injuries are often the first clue to judging their seriousness. Strong forces (such as in a vehicle collision) are likely to cause serious injury.

Head and/or spine injuries should be suspected in any of the following situations:

LOOK OUT FOR...
A serious head injury can occur even if a small child only falls a small distance.

- A fall
- A child found unconscious for unknown reasons
- Any strong blow to the head or trunk
- A sports injury
- Any diving injury
- Any wound to the head or trunk of the body
- Any motor vehicle collision
- Any injury in which the child's helmet is broken
- Electrocution or lightning strike
- Drowning

▶ Prevention

- Keep stairs and other traffic areas clear of toys.
- Use safety gates to keep toddlers off stairs.
- Use childproof latches on windows, cupboards, and balcony doors.
- Ensure crib sides are up whenever you are not within arms' reach.
- Teach children to pick up their toys after play.
- Remove unstable furniture.
- Make sure shelving and doors are secured.
- Put gates at the top and bottom of the stairways.
- Make sure children wear securely fastened running shoes when climbing, running, or playing, especially when on outdoor equipment.
- Make sure that children use appropriate safety equipment when playing sports (e.g., hockey helmets).
- Always wear safety belts and shoulder restraints when driving or riding in a car. Small children must be in approved and properly installed child-restraint systems, such as car seats and booster seats.
- Safety seats must be installed according to the manufacturer's directions. See your nearest public health clinic, police, or fire department for assistance (Figure 8.1).
- Always be careful around water:
  - ▶ enter unknown water feet first
  - ▶ before you dive, make sure the water is deep enough

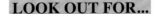

> **LOOK OUT FOR...**
> *Any blow to the nose, jaw, or eye may cause a serious head injury.*

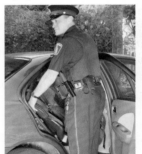

Figure 8.1 Public health clinics, police, or fire departments provide assistance with proper car seat installation.

▶ What to Look For

- Serious headache
- Nausea or vomiting
- Difficulty breathing
- Blood or fluid coming from the ears or nose
- Loss of movement, loss of sensation, or tingling

- Dizziness or disorientation
- Vision problems
- Seizures
- Drowsiness or loss of consciousness
- Swelling, cuts, lumps, and bumps on the head or face

What to Do

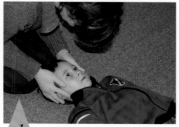

1 Stabilize the head and neck in the position found by holding it with your hands.

2 If the child is wearing a helmet, leave it on unless it makes it difficult for you to manage the ABCs.

NOTE:

Follow the Check, Call, Care steps.

3 If there is blood or clear fluid coming from the nose or ears, do not apply pressure. Lightly dress the area with a clean cloth or gauze and allow the ear to drain.

4 Keep the child calm by comforting and reassuring him.

5 Treat for shock. (See Chapter 4.)

SCALP INJURY

What to Do

- Make sure ABCs are present

NOTE:

Follow the Check, Call, Care steps.

If there doesn't seem to be a fracture:

1 Put dressings on the wound and hold them in place to control the bleeding.

2 Secure the dressings with a bandage.

If you feel a dip, a soft area, or pieces of bone:

NOTE:

If the child has a bump on the head, it is a form of bruise, and ice can be placed on it to reduce swelling.

1 Treat the injury as a head injury.

2 Put direct pressure on the wound only if the bleeding is severe.

3 Try to control the bleeding with pressure on the area around the wound.

4 When performing a secondary survey, pay particular attention to the area of injury because hair may be hiding part of the wound.

SHAKEN BABY SYNDROME (SBS)

SBS happens when people cannot control their anger and frustration when trying to calm a crying and upset baby.

Causes

SBS may happen for several reasons. Sometimes the offender may believe that shaking will help quiet the baby. Some offenders may shake a baby purely out of their own will.

▶ Prevention

- Stay calm. The more frustrated you are, the harder it will be for you to get the baby to settle down.
- If feeding, changing, walking, rocking, and cuddling have not worked, the baby should be gently placed in a safe place and allowed to "cry it out" for a few minutes.
  - ▶ The parent or guardian or caregiver can use the time to relax and calm down before making another attempt to console the baby.
  - ▶ Babysitters should also know that if the above does not work, they should contact the parents or guardians.

▶ What to Look For

- Skull, rib, and long bone fractures
- Bruising, usually on the face or mid-body area
- Bleeding or clear fluid coming from the ears and/or nose
- When do signs and symptoms appear?
  - ▶ Life-threatening injuries take just a few minutes to develop.
  - ▶ Some other symptoms, such as swelling of the brain, can take an average of two to three hours to develop.

What to Do

Injuries suffered from SBS can vary greatly. (See sections throughout this manual for appropriate first aid steps.)

NOTE:

Follow the Check, Call, Care steps.

If you are frustrated, take a break. Never shake.

Modified H.A.IN.E.S. Recovery Position

The modified H.A.IN.E.S. Recovery Position is to be used only if an unconscious person who has a suspected spinal injury must be left alone.

Starting with the person on their back:

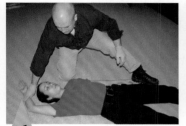

1 Raise the person's arm furthest away from you by rotating it outwards while keeping the palm facing upwards.

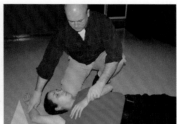

2 Place the arm nearest to you across the chest, with fingers pointing to the opposite shoulder.

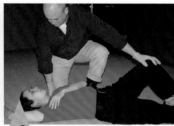

3 Bend the injured person's nearest lower leg at the knee.

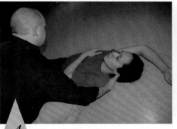

4 Carefully place your forearm nearest to the injured person's head and neck, under the nearest shoulder to provide extra leverage, and to avoid pushing on the head and neck. Place the hand near the head under the hollow of the injured person's neck and head to provide stabilization. DO NOT push or lift the head or neck.

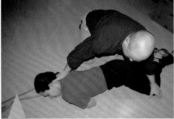

5 Carefully roll the injured person away from yourself by simultaneously pushing on the nearest shoulder, with the forearm of your stabilizing hand, and the flexed knee.

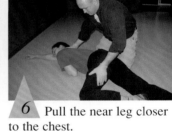

6 Pull the near leg closer to the chest.

NOTE:

Ensure the head remains in contact with the injured person's raised arm and supported by your hand.

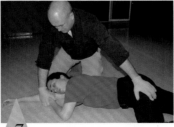

7 Place the hand of the person's upper arm on the outstretched arm against the forehead.

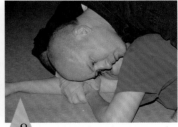

8 Check the airway and, if required, clear with the face turned slightly downwards to permit drainage from the mouth.

Bone, Muscle, and Joint Injuries

You're sitting in the stands at the hockey rink, talking with your neighbour about the upcoming election. You're both hockey parents, and your sons are playing in their semi-finals. You hear a cracking sound and look out onto the ice. Your neighbour's son has just been bodychecked and has fallen on the ice. He's sitting on the ice, crying, and holding his right arm close to his body.

BONE, MUSCLE, AND JOINT INJURIES

There are four basic types of injuries to bones, muscles, and joints:

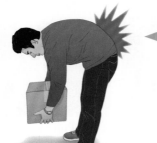

Strain – the stretching or tearing of a muscle or tendon.

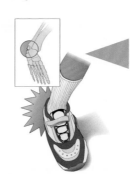

Sprain – the stretching or tearing of ligaments at a joint.

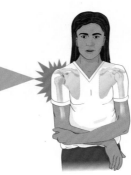

Dislocation – an injury that moves a bone out of its normal position at a joint.

Fracture – a break, chip, or crack in a bone. Fractures can be open, where there is a break in the skin, or closed, where there is no break in the skin.

Causes

- Fall
- Motor vehicle collision
- Sports injury
- Direct blow to the body
- Awkward or sudden movement

Prevention

- Consider the safety of children's everyday activities and environment.
- Ensure children wear seat belts when they're in a vehicle.
- Small children must be in approved and properly installed child-restraint systems, such as car seats or booster seats.
- During activities, make sure children wear the appropriate safety equipment, such as helmets, goggles, and pads.
- When children are bicycling, make sure they always wear a properly fitting, approved helmet (see Chapter 15).
- Put non-slip adhesive strips or mat in the bath.
- Ensure children know the risks and rules of new sports.
- Check the water depth before allowing children to dive.
- Teach children to enter above-ground pools feet first.
- Make sure children stretch before exercising.
- Teach children to know their limits. When they are too tired or frustrated, they should take a break.

What to Look For

- Severe pain or tenderness to the touch
- Deformity or a broken bone sticking out of the skin
- Swelling
- Loss of feeling in a limb
- Discoloration
- The sound of a snap or pop when the injury happened
- Inability to move the body part or difficulty moving it

 ## What to Do

You should call EMS/9-1-1 when:

- The injury involves the head, neck, or back.
- The injury makes walking difficult.

- You suspect that there may be more than one injury.
- There are injuries to the thigh bone or pelvis.
- There is an altered level of consciousness.

If you expect that the ambulance will arrive in a few minutes, keep the child still and do not splint the injury. If the ambulance is going to take longer to arrive, immobilize the injury in the position found using bandages, slings, splints, or blankets.

▶ RICE

General care is the same for all bone, muscle, and joint injuries. You do not need to know the specific injury.

Rest   Avoid any unnecessary movement.

Immobilize   Immobilize the injured area in the position found.

Cold   Apply cold to the injured area. A general rule is 20 minutes every hour for the first 24 to 48 hours. If you use ice, put some sort of thin cloth or pad between it and bare skin to avoid freezing the skin.

Elevation   Elevate the injured area above the level of the heart if possible. However, do not raise the injured area if moving it will cause pain.

▶ Splinting

When using a splint, follow these basic principles:

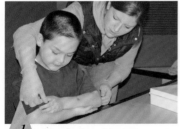

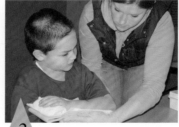

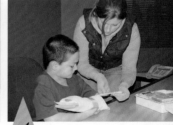

1 Check for skin temperature and colour below the injured area before and after splinting. The area should be warm, indicating good circulation. If the area is cold before splinting, seek medical attention quickly. If the area was warm before splinting and cold afterwards, the splint may be too tight. Loosen it gently.

2 Splint an injury in the position in which you found it.

3 Splint only if you can do it without causing more pain to the child.

4 For joint injuries, splint the bone above and below the injury.

5 For bone injuries, immobilize joints above and below the injury.

There are four types of splints:

- **Soft splints** include folded blankets, towels, pillows, and bandages.

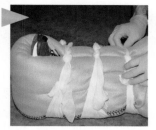

- **Rigid splints** immobilize an injured body part by securing it to something rigid, such as a board, a rolled newspaper, a tree branch, etc.

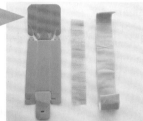

- **Anatomical splints** use another body part for support. For example, you could immobilize an injured leg by securing it to the uninjured leg.

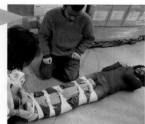

- **Slings** are looped around the neck to support an arm, hand, or wrist.

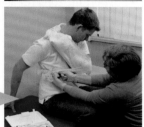

LOOK OUT FOR...

Femur and pelvis fractures are very serious. Do not splint them. Instead, shout for help. Have someone call EMS/9-1-1. If you are alone or no one else can call, you must make the call.

Applying a tube sling for a collarbone fracture:

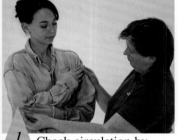

1 Check circulation by checking the fingers for warmth and colour compared to the other limb.
  - Remove any rings the person is wearing.
  - Ask the person if they have any numbness or tingling in the fingers.

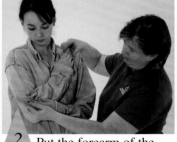

2 Put the forearm of the injured side across the chest, with fingers pointing at the opposite arm.

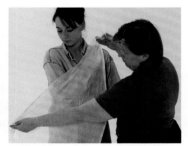

- Position the open triangular bandage over the forearm and hand.
- The point of the triangular bandage should extend past the elbow and shoulder.

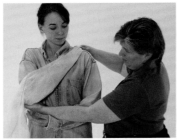

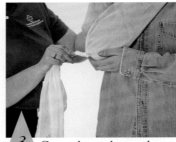

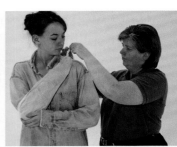

- Support the forearm and carefully tuck the bandage under all the way from the hand to the elbow.

3 Carry the end near the elbow around the back.
- Twist the top of the point of the bandage near the elbow to secure the elbow from coming out of the sling.

- Adjust the height of the sling to make sure it is supporting the arm.
- Tie the ends together in the hollow of the neck on the uninjured side.

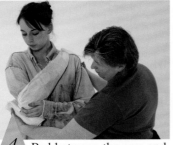

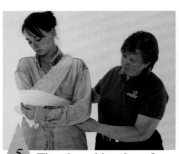

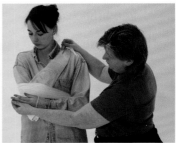

4 Pad between the arm and the body, in the natural hollow, with soft, firm material.

5 Tie a broad bandage from the elbow on the injured side across the body.

Check circulation again for colour or warmth.
- Ask the person if they have any numbness or tingling in the fingers.
- Slings should fit tight enough to restrict movement but not so tight that blood flow is affected.

If the fingers are bluish or cold or if the person feels numbness and tingling, loosen the bandages. If loosening the bandages does not improve circulation, call EMS/9-1-1 immediately.

Wound Care

You're taking the children from the child care centre on a trip to the local fire station. Everyone is excited about seeing the firefighters and their Dalmatian dog. Two of the children are trying to run along the sidewalk, and you are about to stop them. But it's too late. One of them has run right into a parking meter and landed on the ground. Later that afternoon, a huge bruise appears on her left cheek.

WOUNDS

A *wound* is a break in soft tissue. There are two types of wounds: open and closed. A closed wound occurs when there is a break occurring in the tissues under the skin. This is identified by bruising, firmness, and swelling. An open wound is a break in the skin and usually appears as bleeding.

 ### Causes

Wounds are caused by a sudden impact against a part of a person's body. The impact can be from an object that is sharp, heavy, or both.

BRUISES

A *bruise* results from broken blood vessels underneath the skin.

 ### What to Look For

Bruises appear as red or purple blotches or swelling in the skin (Figure 10.1).

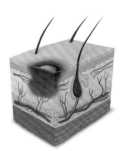

Figure 10.1 A bruise.

 ### What to Do

NOTE:

Follow the Check, Call, Care steps.

1 Elevate the injured part to help reduce swelling.

2 Cool the area to help control both pain and swelling. Apply the cold for 20 minutes every hour. Do this as long as there is pain.

3 When cooling the area, place a cloth or pad between the ice and the skin.

SCRAPES/CUTS

▶ What to Look For

- Bleeding
- Pain
- Skin that is torn away or hanging (Figure 10.2)

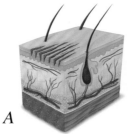 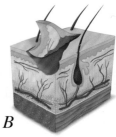

A   B

Figure 10.2 *A*, A scrape.   Figure 10.2 *B*, A cut.

What to Do

> **NOTE:**
>
> *Follow the Check, Call, Care steps.*

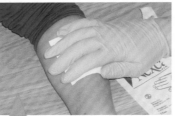

1 If there is much bleeding, put direct pressure on the wound until it stops. If it is a minor wound, wash the wound thoroughly with soap and water.

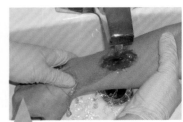

2 Clean the area by rinsing it with water for at least five minutes until the wound shows no sign of foreign matter.

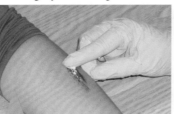

3 Blot the area dry with a sterile gauze dressing and apply antibiotic ointment, only if the parent or guardian of the child has given you permission to do so.

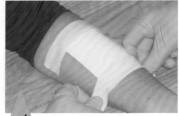

4 Cover the area with a sterile non-stick dressing.

A wound may require stitching if:

- The edges of the skin do not fall together
- The wound is more than 2.5 cm (1 in.) long
- The wound is near joints on the hands or feet
- The wound is on the face

> **NOTE:**
>
> *Wounds should be stitched by a trained medical professional in the first few hours after an injury.*

If the blood soaks through the dressing, add another dressing on top. If you cannot control the bleeding, seek medical attention immediately.

PUNCTURE WOUNDS

Puncture wounds occur when an object pierces the skin but no foreign body remains in the skin. (If an object remains in the skin, this is considered an impaled object; see page 64.)

 Causes

Puncture wounds can be caused by stepping or falling onto a nail, a piece of glass, wood, or other foreign body. Bites are also puncture wounds.

 Prevention

- Develop safe play habits to prevent injury, such as not running with sharp objects.
- Stay away from animals you are unfamiliar with.
- Wear shoes when walking outside.
- Always sweep up broken glass right away.
- Remove nails from boards and dispose of them properly.

 What to Look For

- A hole where the object pierced the skin (Figure 10.3)
- Possible bleeding

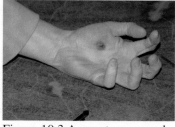

Figure 10.3 A puncture wound.

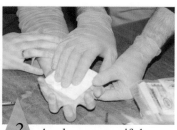 **What to Do**

1. Clean the wound with mild soap and water.

2. Apply pressure if there is bleeding. Dress and bandage the wound.

3. Apply an antibiotic ointment only if the parent or guardian has given permission to do so.

4. Seek medical attention because puncture wounds can be worse than they appear.

5. Watch for signs of infection for the next few days.

> **NOTE:**
>
> *Follow the Check, Call, Care steps.*

BITES FROM HUMANS AND ANIMALS

What to Look For

- Swelling
- Bleeding
- A puncture wound

What to Do

If the bite wound is **bleeding severely**,

1 Apply direct pressure with a clean cloth.

2 Call EMS/9-1-1.

3 Comfort the child and keep her warm.

If the bite wound is **not bleeding severely**,

NOTE:

Follow the Check, Call, Care steps.

1 Wash with a mild soap and water.

2 Cover the wound with a sterile dressing. Bandage the dressing in place. Then seek medical attention.

3 Comfort the child and keep her warm.

4 Watch for signs of infection for the next few days.

▶ Notes on Animal and Human Bites

- For animal bites, have someone note the location of the animal. It should be captured by animal control for examination.
- Human bites can easily become infected. Be especially careful to wash with soap and water and follow up by seeking medical attention.

AMPUTATIONS

An *amputation* is a complete severing of a body part. Although there is damage to the tissues, bleeding is usually not deadly (Figure 10.4).

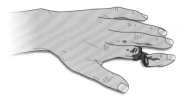

Figure 10.4 An amputation.

▶ Cause

An amputation may be caused by any force great enough to completely or partially cut or tear away a limb from the rest of the body.

▶ Prevention

- Ensure that children's hands are clear from all doors when closing.
- Do not allow children to play on or near train tracks.
- Teach children not to put their fingers near the spokes of a moving bicycle tire.
- Farm machinery causes many serious injuries. Do not allow children to play on or near any farm machinery, even when it is turned off.

▶ What to Look For

- Shock
- A part of the body completely or partially disconnected from the rest of the body
- Pain
- Bleeding

What to Do

1 Treat any bleeding with direct pressure.

2 Shout for help. Have someone call EMS/9-1-1. If alone, you must make the call.

NOTE:
Remember your gloves and other barrier devices.

3 Try to retrieve the amputated body part.

4 Wrap the amputated part in a clean cloth.

NOTE:
Follow the Check, Call, Care steps.

5 Place the amputated part in a plastic bag.

John Smith
25/03/06
1:35pm

6 Keep the amputated part cool by placing the bag on ice. Don't put the part directly on ice as it will freeze.

7 Label the container that contains the body part (child's name, date, and time).

8 Make sure the amputated part goes with the injured child to the hospital.

9 Comfort the child and keep her warm.

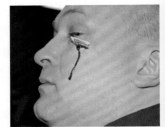

Figure 10.5 An impaled object.

IMPALED OBJECTS

An *impaled object* is a foreign object that is sticking out from the skin or eye (Figure 10.5).

▶ **Causes**

Impalement can be caused by falling onto something sharp such as scissors or broken glass or falling while carrying something sharp, such as a knife.

▶ **Prevention**

See prevention for puncture wounds.

▶ **What to Look For**

- Pain
- A foreign object sticking out of the skin
- Bleeding

▶ **What to Do**

1 Call EMS/9-1-1 if the impaled object is large or if it is impaled in the head, neck, or torso.

2 Expose the area around the wound. Cut clothing away from the wound area instead of pulling clothing over it.

3 Leave the impaled object in place unless it is in the way of treating any life-threatening injuries. If there is a life-threatening injury, call EMS/9-1-1.

6 Seek medical attention if EMS/9-1-1 hasn't already been called.

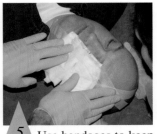

4 Stabilize the impaled object by putting bulky dressings around it.

5 Use bandages to keep the dressings in place.

NOSEBLEEDS

▶ Causes

- Forceful nose blowing
- Nose picking
- Trauma to the nose
- Dry weather conditions
- High blood pressure
- Bleeding disorders

▶ Prevention

- Use a humidifier if the air indoors is dry.
- Wear protective athletic equipment when participating in sports that could cause injury to the nose.
- Encourage gentle nose blowing.
- Teach children not to pick their nose.

▶ What to Look For

- Blood coming from the nose

NOTE:
Follow the Check, Call, Care steps.

What to Do

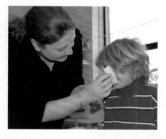

1 Have the child sit down.

2 Tilt the child's head forward slightly.

3 Pinch the nose firmly between the bone and the tip of the nose.

4 Hold firmly for 10 minutes.

LOOK OUT FOR...

If bleeding continues, call EMS/9-1-1, allow the nose to drain, and place the child in the recovery position. (See Chapter 4.)

5 Seek medical attention unless you are aware that this is a common occurrence for the child.

FOREIGN OBJECTS IN THE EYE

▶ Causes

Can be caused by dirt, dust, sand, or other debris entering the eye

▶ What to Look For

- Foreign objects in the eye, such as particles of dirt, sand, embers, glass, metal, or an impaled object

- A scratchy feeling when blinking or with eye movement
- Watering of the eye

 What to Do

1 Wash hands before examining the eye.

NOTE:

Follow the Check, Call, Care steps.

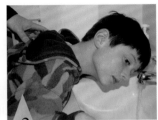

2 With the head tilted and the affected eye towards the ground, flush the eye, from the nose to the outside of head, using water from a clean pitcher or by running water from a tap.

3 If the object appears to be impaled, do not attempt to dislodge it.

4 Seek medical attention.

LOOK OUT FOR...

If there is an impaled object in the eye, call EMS/9-1-1.

FOREIGN OBJECT IN THE EAR

▶ **What to Look For**

- A tiny object, such as a bean, pea, button, or seed
- An insect

 What to Do

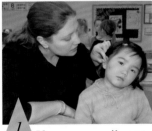

1 If you can easily see and grasp the object, remove it.

2 Tilt the head to the affected side and gently tap above the ear to see if the object falls out.

NOTE:

Follow the Check, Call, Care steps.

3 If the object does not dislodge easily, leave the object in place for a medical professional to remove. Trying to remove the object by using a pin, toothpick, or similar sharp object could force the object further back. You could also puncture the ear drum.

FOREIGN OBJECTS IN THE NOSE

▶ **What to Look For**

- Stuffy-sounding nose
- Nose deformity
- Bleeding
- An object in the nose
- Unusually bad breath (if the object has been there for a while)

What to Do

1 If the child is in great pain or has difficulty breathing, call EMS/9-1-1.

2 Keep the child from digging for the object with her finger.

3 Try to prevent the child from blowing her nose.

4 If you can easily see and grasp the object, remove it.

5 If the object does not dislodge easily, leave it in place for a medical professional to remove. Trying to remove the object by using a pin, toothpick, or similar sharp object could force the object further into the nose.

NOTE:

Follow the Check, Call, Care steps.

KNOCKED-OUT TEETH

► Cause

Any kind of blow or fall that involves the mouth

► Prevention

• Wear appropriate equipment when playing sports, such as a mouth guard or face mask.

• Always wear a seat belt while in the car and do not eat or drink in a moving car.

► What to Look For

• Loose or dislodged teeth
• Possible head or spine injury (see Chapter 8)
• Bleeding
• Swelling

NOTE:

Follow the Check, Call, Care steps.

What to Do

1 Ensure that the injured child's airway is open. (See Chapter 5.)

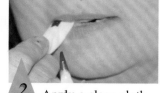

2 Apply a clean cloth or dressing to bleeding areas and have the child bite down on it.

► Ensure that blood can drain away from any bleeding areas and that the child will not swallow the dressing.

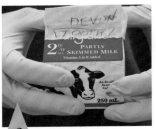

 4 Apply cold to any swelling.

5 Get the child and the tooth to a dentist as soon as possible. The greatest chance of repair is during the first hour after the tooth was knocked out.

3 Place the broken tooth in milk. Hold the tooth by the crown only and avoid touching the cracked edge or the root. If there is no milk, put the tooth in water or wrap it in a clean cloth. Seal the container and label it with the child's name, date, and time.

NOTE:
Consider how the injury happened and treat for a head injury if necessary. (See Chapter 8.)

SPLINTERS (SLIVERS)

▶ Description

A ***splinter*** (sliver) is a small piece of wood, metal, or other material embedded into the skin.

 What to Do

1 If the splinter is sticking out of the skin, use tweezers to pull it out. Pull out at the same angle that the splinter entered the skin.

2 If the splinter is difficult to remove, call the parents/guardians and allow them to deal with it.

3 Keep the wound clean and watch for signs of infection for a few days.

INFECTION

Infection occurs when organisms, such as bacteria or viruses, enter the body and the body's own immune system is unable to destroy them.

▶ Causes

Infection is caused by dirt, foreign bodies, or bacteria present in a wound (Figure 10.6).

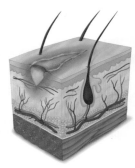

Figure 10.6 An infection.

▶ Prevention

- Ensure that all wounds are kept clean and bandaged properly. Prevention is the best defence against infection.
- Keep immunizations up to date.
- Wash your hands often.

▶ What to Look For

- Swelling, redness, and warmth around the wound
- Pain in the area of the wound
- Sometimes pus discharge

A more serious infection may cause the following symptoms:

- Fever
- Feeling nauseated
- Red streaks that progress from the wound towards the heart

> **NOTE:**
> *Seek medical attention if an infection is suspected.*

BURNS

Burns are injuries caused by chemicals, electricity, heat, or radiation.

Table 10.1 *Seriousness of Burns*

Types	What to Look for	What to Do
Superficial burns	• Redness • Pain • Possible swelling	• Cool with running or standing water until pain stops (possibly about 10–20 minutes). If the standing water becomes warm, add more cool water. • Once the burning has stopped, you can apply an antibiotic ointment but only if parents have given permission to do so. Watch for signs of infection.
Partial-thickness burns	• Redness • Pain • Possible swelling • Blisters	• If the burned area covers more than 10% of the child's body, call EMS/9-1-1 and treat the child for shock. Cool only a small area at a time. Cooling the child too quickly may cause the child to go into shock. • If the burned area covers less than 10% of the child's body, cool the burn with standing water for at least 10–20 minutes. If this is too painful or the area cannot be put in water, cover the burn with a cool, moist sterile dressing or clean cloth to cool it. • Only remove jewellery and/or clothing that is not stuck to the skin. • After cooling the skin, cover it loosely with a dry, sterile dressing, preferably non-stick gauze. • Seek medical attention.

Types	What to Look for	What to Do
Full-thick-ness burn	• Red • Painful at the edges of the burn. Possible nerve damage may cause the burn to be non-painful. • May swell • Blisters • Charred or waxy white flesh • Open wound	• Call EMS/9-1-1. • If the burned area covers more than 10% of the child's body, treat the child for shock. Cool only a small area at a time. Cooling the child too quickly may cause the child to go into shock. • If the burned area covers less than 10% of the child's body, cool the burn with standing water. If this is too painful or the area cannot be put in water, cover the burn with a cool, moist sterile dressing or clean cloth to cool it. • Only remove jewellery and/or clothing that is not stuck to the skin. • Do not try to clean a full-thickness burn. • After cooling the skin, cover it loosely with a dry, sterile dressing, preferably non-stick gauze. • Treat for shock.

Table 10.2 *Types of Burns*

Types	Prevention	What To Do
Chemical burns	• Store chemicals in their original containers. • Keep chemicals out of reach of children. • Put locking devices on cupboards that contain chemicals. • Make sure that your child care facility has been set up according to the Workplace Hazardous Materials Information System (WHMIS), health and safety regulations, and any other regulatory bodies governing your facility.	• Call EMS/9-1-1. • Brush off excess dry chemicals. Be careful not to get the chemical on your own body. • Flush with large amounts of free-flowing water for at least 15 minutes. • Remove any chemical-soaked clothing from the injured child.

Types	Prevention	What To Do
Electrical burns	• Keep electrical appliances away from water. • Repair or discard frayed cords. • Use protective outlet plates.	• Call EMS/9-1-1. • Touch the injured child only after the power source has been removed. • Check the ABCs (airway, breathing, circulation). • Treat as a head and spine injury. (See Chapter 8.) • Look for two burns, an entry point and an exit point. Entry and exit points will need to be treated as open wounds.
Heat burns	• Keep matches away from children. • Keep storage areas free of clutter and store all flammable materials safely. • Keep children away from any cooking appliances when they are in use. • Stay by the stove when stove elements or the oven is turned on. • Keep hot tea and coffee out of reach of children. • Keep the hot water tank temperature turned down to 49°C (120°F) or use anti-scald devices on taps.	• Care for the injured child according to the level of burn. (See Table 10.1 on page 70.)

Types	Prevention	What To Do
Sunburns	• Limit exposure to the sun during the time between 10:00 a.m. and 3:00 p.m. • Ensure that children wear proper clothing to prevent overexposure. • If given permission by the parent or guardian, use sunscreen with a sun protection factor (SPF) of at least 25. Reapply at least every two hours and after being in the water or after vigorous activity or sweating.	• Care for the injured child according to the level of burn. (See Table 10.1 on page 70.)

▶ Special Considerations for All Types of Burns

• For large-area burns, apply cold to only a small area at a time.

• Keep any fabric or clothing that is stuck to the skin in place.

• Only use ice or ice water on a small area of a superficial burn. If ice or ice water is used, use only for 10 minutes.

• Resist the urge to break blisters.

• Cover a burn only with a clean or sterile dressing. Use a non-stick dressing if available.

• If more than 10% of the body's surface area is burned, do not attempt to cool the burns. This may lower the injured child's body temperature.

• Seek immediate medical attention for serious burns or if the burn involves large areas of the head, face, hands, feet, or groin.

• Use ointments only on superficial burns. A doctor or pharmacist can recommend what product to use.

Sudden Medical Emergencies

You are standing in line outside the ice-cream parlour after seeing a movie with your seven-year-old son. It's about 3 p.m., and you've been waiting for about 20 minutes. Your son suddenly slumps to the ground.

FAINTING

Fainting results in a loss of consciousness. It is caused by a temporary lack of blood flow to the brain.

▶ **Causes**

- Dehydration
- Pain
- Heat
- Stress or fear
- Standing for long periods of time
- Low blood sugar
- High fever

▶ **What to Look For**

Fainting may be preceded by:

- Paleness
- Sweating
- Dizziness
- Nausea

 What to Do

△ *1* If you think that a child is about to faint, have him lie down.

△ *2* If the child does faint, place him in the recovery position. (See Chapter 4.) Then watch his breathing closely.

△ *3* As he awakens, keep him at rest and warm.

△ *4* If the child does not awaken within a minute, call EMS/9-1-1.

DIABETES

To function, the body uses sugar as a source of energy. To use sugar, the body needs insulin, which it normally makes itself. If the body does not make enough insulin or does not use it properly, the person has **diabetes**.

▶ Causes

Diabetic emergencies are caused by an imbalance in a person's sugar and insulin levels.

▶ Prevention

- If the child is a known diabetic, he should wear a MedicAlert® medical identification product.
- Take any medications as prescribed.
- Keep quick-sugar foods with you at all times.

> **NOTE:**
> *Not all children with a blood sugar emergency are diabetic.*

▶ What to Look For

- Changes in the level of consciousness
- Rapid breathing
- Confusion or aggression
- A MedicAlert® medical identification product.
- Pale, cool, sweaty skin

What to Do

If the diabetic child is conscious:

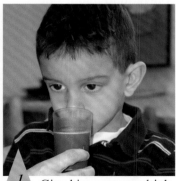

1 Give him a sugary drink, such as orange or apple juice.

2 His condition should improve within 5 minutes. If there is no improvement, call EMS/9-1-1.

> **NOTE:**
> *Follow the Check, Call, Care steps.*

> **NOTE:**
> *You do not need to know the different types of diabetic emergencies because the treatment is always the same.*

If the diabetic child is unconscious:

 1 Call EMS/9-1-1.

2 Check ABCs (airway, breathing, and circulation).

3 Place him in the recovery position. (See Chapter 4.)

4 Treat for shock. (See Chapter 4.)

SEIZURES

Seizures can take many forms. Some are severe, uncontrolled muscle spasms, whereas others can take the form of unusual sensations or changes in behaviour.

 ### Causes

All seizures result from an interruption of electrical activity in the brain. This interruption in activity may be caused by:

- Head injuries
- Poisons
- Fever
- Infection
- Some medical conditions, such as epilepsy and diabetes
- Certain video games or other audiovisual stimulation that involves flashes

Prevention

- Follow the guidelines throughout this book for preventing injuries at work, home, or play.
- If you have epilepsy, take your prescribed medication regularly.
- If your child has a fever, make sure it doesn't get too high. If a child's fever is higher than a fever caused by a normal cold or flu, see a doctor.
- Limit the amount of time spent playing video games.

 ### What to Look For

- Eyes may roll upwards, back into the head
- Signs of drooling or foam in the mouth
- A sense of urgency to get to safety

- Hallucinations, such as seeing, hearing, tasting, or smelling something that doesn't actually exist
- Appearance of daydreaming
- Uncontrollable muscle movement

  What to Do

> **NOTE:**
>
> *Follow the Check, Call, Care steps.*

 1 Call EMS/9-1-1.

2 Protect the child's head and limbs from injury by removing nearby objects.

3 Place pillows or other soft objects between the child's head and immovable objects, such as walls and heavy furniture.

4 Allow the child to move without restraint.

5 Keep all objects away from the child's mouth.

6 After the seizure, place the child in the recovery position. (See Chapter 4.)

7 Check ABCs.

8 Comfort the child. Keep him warm.

> **NOTE:**
>
> *Some temper tantrums may look like seizures. This would be the case if the child holds her breath or hyperventilates to the point of fainting. However, a child who loses consciousness in a tantrum will automatically begin breathing again. This is not the case in a seizure.*

If the child is a known epileptic, follow the directions of the parents or guardians or doctor as to when to call EMS/9-1-1. Generally, you will need to call EMS/9-1-1 for any of the following reasons:

- The seizure lasts longer than five minutes.
- The child is injured during the seizure.
- He does not wake up after the seizure is over.
- The seizure takes place in water.
- There are repeated succeeding seizure episodes.

Chapter *12*

Environmental Emergencies

A father and his 11-year-old daughter go ice fishing early one Saturday morning. It's a sunny day, and they stay out longer than planned. By lunchtime, his daughter is shivering, but she warms up over a fire. As they start packing to leave, the daughter wanders away to look at another hole in the ice and falls right in. By the time her father gets her to land, she is numb and confused.

FROST NIP/FROSTBITE

Frost nip is a superficial freezing of the skin. In a case of *frostbite*, the tissue and fluids underneath the skin freeze and swell.

▶ Cause

- Exposure to cold temperatures

▶ Prevention

- Avoid exposing any part of the body to cold or frozen objects.
- Wear appropriate clothing. For example, wear a hat and layers of clothing made of tightly woven fibres, such as wool. These trap warm air against your body.
- Keep vulnerable areas such as fingers, toes, ears, and nose covered with warm clothing.

▶ What to Look For

Frost nip (Figure 12.1) has the following symptoms:

- Pain or stinging in the affected area, followed by numbness
- Area on the skin that looks paler than the area around it

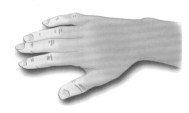

Figure 12.1 Frost nip.

If conditions worsen, **frostbite** (Figure 12.2) may develop. Frostbite has these symptoms:

- Skin is pale, waxy, flushed, yellow, or blue.
- Skin is hard or solid and cold to the touch.
- There is numbness or a lack of feeling in the affected area.
- Blisters may be present after thawing.

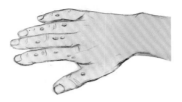

Figure 12.2 Frostbite.

What to Do

NOTE:
Follow the Check, Call, Care steps.

△ *1* Remove the injured child from the cold environment.

△ *2* Use warm water or body heat to gradually warm the affected area.

△ *3* Leave blisters and protect with loose, dry dressings.

△ *4* If frostbite is suspected, seek medical attention.

Do not rub or apply snow to a frost-nipped or frostbitten body part.

Rewarm a frost nipped or frostbitten part only if you are sure it will not refreeze.

HYPOTHERMIA

Hypothermia is a life-threatening condition. It develops when the body temperature drops too low. This is usually because the child has been out in the cold too long.

- Hypothermia can be mild, moderate, or severe.
- Hypothermia can get worse very quickly if the child is wet in a cold environment.
- Hypothermia can get worse slowly if the child is dry but the environment is cold.
- Hypothermia can occur at any time of the year.

 Prevention

Hypothermia can usually be prevented with common sense and by following these guidelines:

- Keep children indoors during the coldest part of the day. Each province or territory has regulations as to when children are not to be taken outdoors.

- Make sure children wear hats and layers of clothing made of tightly woven fibres, which trap warm air against the body. (Wool is a good example.)
- Have children drink plenty of warm fluids. This will help keep the body at a normal temperature.
- If hot drinks are not available, provide plenty of plain water.
- As soon as shivering starts, get children out of the cold. Let their bodies warm up. This will help get them through brief times of extreme cold.
- When near water, ensure that children are careful not to fall in.
- Have children change out of wet clothing as soon as they come in from the cold. Have them put on warm, dry clothing.

Table 12.1 *Hypothermia: Levels of Severity*

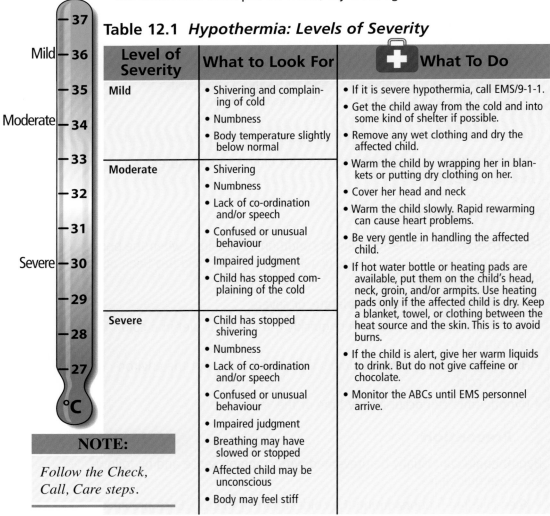

	Level of Severity	What to Look For	What To Do
Mild	Mild	• Shivering and complaining of cold • Numbness • Body temperature slightly below normal	• If it is severe hypothermia, call EMS/9-1-1. • Get the child away from the cold and into some kind of shelter if possible. • Remove any wet clothing and dry the affected child.
Moderate	Moderate	• Shivering • Numbness • Lack of co-ordination and/or speech • Confused or unusual behaviour • Impaired judgment • Child has stopped complaining of the cold	• Warm the child by wrapping her in blankets or putting dry clothing on her. • Cover her head and neck • Warm the child slowly. Rapid rewarming can cause heart problems. • Be very gentle in handling the affected child. • If hot water bottle or heating pads are available, put them on the child's head, neck, groin, and/or armpits. Use heating pads only if the affected child is dry. Keep a blanket, towel, or clothing between the heat source and the skin. This is to avoid burns.
Severe	Severe	• Child has stopped shivering • Numbness • Lack of co-ordination and/or speech • Confused or unusual behaviour • Impaired judgment • Breathing may have slowed or stopped • Affected child may be unconscious • Body may feel stiff	• If the child is alert, give her warm liquids to drink. But do not give caffeine or chocolate. • Monitor the ABCs until EMS personnel arrive.

Temperature scale (°C): 37, 36 (Mild), 35, 34 (Moderate), 33, 32, 31, 30 (Severe), 29, 28, 27

NOTE:

Follow the Check, Call, Care steps.

FREEZING OF SKIN TO METAL OBJECTS

Children sometimes cannot resist licking ice from fences and other metal objects. They may be dared to do this. They may just be curious. Whatever the reason, the result is painful.

What to Look For

- Child's skin or tongue is stuck to a metal object

What to Do

△ *1* Apply warm (not hot) water to the surface of the object and/or the skin that is stuck to the object.

△ *2* Gradually and gently help release the child.

△ *3* Treat the torn skin as an open wound. (See Chapter 10.)

△ *4* Reassure and calm the child.

SNOW BLINDNESS

Snow blindness is caused by overexposure to the sun's ultraviolet (UV) rays. A child is at higher risk than an adult because the lens in a child's eye does not block UV rays as well as the lens in an adult's eye.

▶ Prevention

- Have children wear sunglasses with at least 99% UV protection. This provides protection from the sun's UV rays.
- Install blinds that can be opened and closed to regulate sunlight entering your home or child care setting, for example, venetian or roller blinds.

▶ What to Look For

- Redness
- Burning sensation
- Swelling
- Pain in the eyes

What to Do

△ *1* Cool, damp cloths on the eyes may ease pain and burning.

△ *2* Seek medical attention.

HEAT-RELATED EMERGENCIES

Heat-related emergencies occur when the body's temperature gets too high. Heat cramps, heat exhaustion, and heat stroke are all head-related emergencies.

 Causes

Heat-related emergencies may be caused by the following:

- Too much time spent in the heat or sun
- Not drinking enough. This means that fluids lost by sweating are not replaced.
- Exercising too hard in hot weather

 Prevention

Most heat-related emergencies can be prevented with common sense and the following guidelines:

- Keep children indoors during the hottest part of the day. Each province or territory has regulations as to when children are not to be taken outdoors.
- Make sure children slow down their activities as it gets hotter.
- Ensure that children take frequent breaks in a cool or shaded area. This way their bodies will cool off and be able to withstand brief periods of heat exposure.
- Have children dress for the heat and their activity level.
- Make sure children wear a hat when in the sun. They should also wear light-coloured cotton clothing to absorb sweat. Their clothing should also let air circulate and heat escape.
- Ensure that children drink plenty of cool fluids. Do not use drinks with caffeine. Drinking plenty of fluids is the most important way to prevent heat emergencies.

Table 12.2 *Heat-Related Emergencies*

Type of Injury	What to Look For	What To Do
Heat cramps	• Mild muscle contractions that may become severe, usually in the legs and abdomen • Body temperature usually normal • Moist skin	1. Have the child rest in a cool place. 2. Provide fluids, preferably juices or sports drinks appropriate for children. 3. Gently stretch and massage the muscles involved. **NOTE:** *Follow the Check, Call, Care steps.*

Heat exhaustion	• Normal or slightly elevated body temperature
	
	• Cool, moist, pale or red skin
	
	• Nausea
	
	• Dizziness and weakness
	
	• Exhaustion
		1. Have the child rest in a cool place.
		2. Loosen any tight clothing. Remove clothing soaked with sweat.
		3. Put cool water on the skin and fan the child to increase evaporation.
		4. If the child is conscious, have her take sips of cool water.
		5. Check and record vital signs on a regular basis. (See Chapter 4.)
		   • The child should not return to activities in the heat on this day.
		   • If the condition worsens, treat for heat stroke (see below).

Heat stroke	• High body temperature, often as high as 41°C (106°F) • Red, hot, dry skin • Irritable, bizarre, or combative behaviour • Progressive loss of consciousness • Seizures • Rapid, shallow breathing	1. Call EMS/9-1-1. 2. Have the child rest in a cool place. 3. Sponge the entire body with tepid or cool water; fan the child. Use ice packs or cold packs. Place them in the groin, in each armpit, and on the neck to cool large blood vessels. Be careful not to place them directly on the skin.

47
46
45
44
43
42
41 Heat Stroke
40
39
38 Heat Exhaustion
37 Heat Cramps
°C

Chapter 13

Poisons

You are taking the children for a nature walk through a meadow. The August sun is shining, and bees are feeding from the asters and goldenrod. One of the boys goes to sniff the flowers but gets a bee sting instead. He jumps up and down in pain, upsetting other bees and getting stung again.

POISONS

A *poison* is a substance that may be harmless in some instances but when introduced to the body, it causes injury, illness, or death. Poisons may include drugs, medicines, plants, and dozens of common household cleaning products.

A poison can enter the body by being:

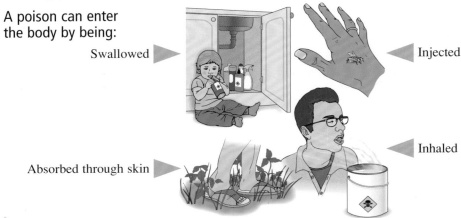

Swallowed

Injected

Absorbed through skin

Inhaled

▶ Prevention

Follow these general guidelines to help prevent poisoning:

LOOK OUT FOR...

The most common poison among children is non-prescription medication.

- Keep all medications, household products, poisonous plants, and other substances well out of the reach of children.
- Use locked cupboards or special child-resistant latches.
- Consider all household or drugstore products as potentially harmful.
- Use child-resistant safety caps on medications and other products.
- Never call medicine "candy" to entice a child to take it.

- Keep products in their original containers with labels.
- Use poison symbols to identify dangerous substances. Teach children what these symbols mean.
- Carefully dispose of outdated and poisonous products. Do not dispose of them in places where children can access them.
- Keep the telephone number of your local Poison Control Centre beside your telephone at home, at the workplace, and at child care centres.

HAZARD SYMBOLS

When any of the following symbols appear on a container, the contents are dangerous. They must therefore be stored appropriately.

Table 13.1 *The Hazard Symbols*

Explosive The container can explode if heated or punctured. Flying pieces of metal or plastic from the container can cause serious injury, especially to eyes.	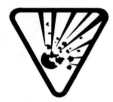
Corrosive The product can burn your skin or eyes. If swallowed, it will damage your throat and stomach.	
Flammable The product or its fumes will catch fire easily if it is near heat, flames or sparks. Rags used with this product may begin to burn on their own.	
Poison If you swallow, lick, or, in some cases, breathe in the chemical, you could become very sick or die.	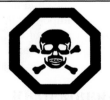

REMEMBER:

Approach the child only if the area is safe. If it is not safe, call EMS/9-1-1.

EMS/9-1-1 OR POISON CONTROL CENTRE

Poison Control Centre
Telephone Number _____

The ABCs (airway, breathing, and circulation) will tell you how to respond to all types of poisoning.

- If the child is conscious and alert and the ABCs are fine, call your local Poison Control Centre.

- If the child has an altered level of consciousness or has difficulty breathing, call EMS/9-1-1.

SWALLOWED POISONS

Swallowed poisons are poisons that enter the body by contact with the mouth or lips.

 What to Look For

- Product residue in the affected area
- Abdominal cramps and vomiting
- Unconsciousness
- A burning sensation in the mouth, throat, or stomach

- Burns around the mouth
- Seizures
- Dizziness and/or drowsiness

 What to Do

NOTE:

Follow the Check, Call, Care steps.

LOOK OUT FOR...

Never induce vomiting if the child is unconscious, is having seizures, or has swallowed a corrosive or petroleum product.

1 If the Poison Control Centre advises you to do so, have someone drive you and the child to the hospital. It is important that you carefully monitor the child. Take a sample of the poison and any vomit with the child to the hospital.

3 Give water or milk or induce vomiting only if directed to do so by the Poison Control Centre.

2 Look at the packaging of the substance if available. This may help you find out what the poison is.

4 Monitor ABCs (airway, breathing, and circulation).

5 Treat for shock. (See Chapter 4.)

INHALED POISONS

Inhaled poisons are poisons that are breathed into the body.

▶ **What to Look For**

- Breathing difficulties
- Dizziness
- Seizures
- Bluish colour around the mouth
- Cloud in the air

- Irritated eyes, nose, throat
- Vomiting
- Unusual smell
- Unconsciousness

 What to Do

If the child is conscious:

1 Protect yourself from the poison.

2 Get the affected child to fresh air immediately.

NOTE:
Follow the Check, Call, Care steps.

If the child is unconscious:

1 Protect yourself from the poison.

2 Get the affected child to fresh air immediately if it is safe for you to do so.

3 If the child is not breathing, start CPR. (See Chapter 7.) Remember to use a barrier device so that you don't contaminate yourself with the poison.

4 Treat for shock. (See Chapter 4.)

ABSORBED POISONS

Absorbed poisons are poisons that go through the skin. They are often chemicals or poisons found in plants.

▶ **What to Look For**

- Burns
- Rash
- Itching
- Blisters
- Unconsciousness

- Fever
- Burning
- Swelling
- Hives

What to Do

1 Be sure that you are wearing protective clothing.

2 Remove the poisonous substance from the skin.

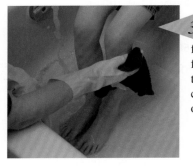

3 Flush the area with water for 20 minutes. Flush away from the rest of the body so that the poison does not come in contact with more of the body.

4 Monitor ABCs (airway, breathing, and circulation).

INJECTED POISONS

Injected poisons are poisons that enter the body through bites or stings or as a drug injected with a needle.

▶ Prevention

When in wooded or grassy areas, follow these general guidelines to prevent poisoning through bites from insects and ticks.

- Children should wear long-sleeved shirts and pants.
- They should tuck their pant legs into their socks or boots and tuck their shirt into their pants.
- Have children wear light-coloured but not bright clothing. This makes it easier to see tiny insects or ticks.
- They should not wear perfume or other scents.
- In tick-infested areas, use a rubber band or tape to close off the area where children's pants and socks meet. This way nothing can get under their clothing.
- When hiking in woods and fields, keep children in the middle of trails.
- Make sure children avoid underbrush and tall grass.
- Inspect children carefully for insects or ticks after they've been outdoors.
- Inspect children for leeches after they've come out of a water source, such as a lake.

BITES AND STINGS FROM INSECTS

▶ What to Look For

- Itching and pain in the affected area
- Swelling or redness in the affected area

> **NOTE:**
>
> *Follow the Check, Call, Care steps.*

 What to Do

1 Find out if the child is known to be sensitive to stings. If he has an epinephrine auto-injector, help him use it.

2 Rinse the affected area. Remove the stinger by gently scraping it out. Squeezing the stinger may inject more poison, so don't use tweezers.

3 Apply a cold compress to the area to control swelling. Do this for 20 minutes every hour.

4 Treat for shock.

BITES FROM TICKS

▶ What to Look For

- Tick is on or embedded in the skin
  - Area around the tick is red or swollen

 What to Do

1 Remove the tick with tweezers if it has started to dig into the skin.

- Grasp it as close to the skin as possible.
- Pull slowly.
- If you do not have tweezers, use a glove, plastic wrap, or a piece of paper to protect your fingers.

2 Wash your hands immediately.

3 Treat the torn skin as an open wound. (See Chapter 10.)

4 Reassure and calm the child.

> **NOTE:**
>
> *If the tick is on the skin, remove it by brushing it off.*

5 If you have been given permission by a parent or guardian, use an antibiotic ointment to prevent infection. If a rash or flu-like symptoms occur later, seek medical attention.

- Do not try to burn off the tick.
- Do not coat the tick with petroleum jelly or nail polish.
- Do not prick the tick with a pin.
- Avoid twisting or squeezing the tick.

LYME DISEASE

Lyme disease is caused by a bite from an infected tick.

 What to Look For

Early symptoms:

- A rash in a small red area that spreads up to 13–18 cm (5–7 in.) across
- Fever, headache, weakness, and joint and muscle pain that may feel like the flu

Later symptoms, which may appear weeks or months after the bite:

- Arthritis, numbness, or a stiff neck
- Memory loss
- Problems seeing or hearing
- A high fever
- An irregular or rapid heartbeat

 What to Do

Seek medical attention.

BITES FROM LEECHES (BLOOD SUCKERS)

What to Look For

- A leech is still stuck to the skin

 What to Do

1 Sprinkle with salt. Then remove the leech.

2 Wash the wound area with soap and water.

3 Watch for signs of infection, redness, swelling, or pain at the injury site.

Childhood Illnesses

When you babysit your neighbour's two daughters, they usually want to run around the yard, draw pictures, or play house. But this October evening, the eight-year-old is moody and doesn't feel like doing anything. You notice that she looks pale and her skin is warm.

RECOGNIZING SIGNS OF ILLNESS

If you are a child care worker and you think a child under your care may be ill, ask the parents or guardians:

• How did your child sleep last night?

• How has she been eating and drinking?

• What is her mood?

As a child care worker, parent, or guardian, ask yourself the following questions.

Table 14.1 *Questions to Ask Yourself If You Think a Child May Be Ill*

Area to Watch	Questions
Behaviour	Is the child… • Confused? • Unusually sleepy? • Unusually irritable or fussy? • Not interested in eating or drinking? • More active or more subdued than normal? • Not interested in other children or play? • Crying nonstop, even when cuddled?
Face	Does the child… • Appear pale or flushed? • Show signs of pain or anxiety? • Have bluish lips?

Area to Watch	Questions
Skin	Does the child have… • Warm and dry or cold and moist skin? • A rash or spots? • An unusual skin colour? • Itchy skin? • Any bruising or swelling?
Eyes	Does the child… • Rub and scratch her eyes? • Squint? • Have red and inflamed eyes? • Have discharge in her eyes? • Have dull or unusually bright eyes? • Have swollen or puffy eyes? • Have yellow eyes? • Complain of seeing spots?
Ears	Does the child have… • Trouble hearing? • Swelling? • Ringing in the ears? • An ear ache? • Any discharge? • Loss of balance? • A tendency to pull, cup, or poke her ears?
Tongue	Does the child have a… • Dry and cracked tongue? • Red and raw tongue? • White or yellow coating on her tongue?
Breath	Does the child have a… • Strange odour on her breath?
Breathing	Does the child have… • Rapid shallow breathing? • Painful breathing?

Area to Watch	Questions
Throat	Does the child have… • Pain? • Difficulty swallowing? • Unusual drooling? • A red and inflamed throat? • A voice that sounds different?
Cough	Does the cough… • Occur frequently, and is it dry? • Bring up sputum?
Appetite	Does the child have… • A lost appetite? • An unusual craving for certain types of food?
Vomiting	Is the child… • Unable to keep food or water down? • Nauseated? • Frequently vomiting? • Projectile vomiting?
Temperature	Does the child… • Complain about feeling very cold? • Complain about feeling very hot? • Shiver uncontrollably?
Bowel movements	Are the child's bowel movements… • Abnormally frequent and liquid? • Abnormally infrequent, dry, and hard? • Abnormal in content, such as undigested food, mucus, or blood? • An unusual colour or odour?

14.2 *Childhood Conditions*

Condition	What to Look For	🩹 What to Do	Remember
Eczema Not contagious **Note:** Eczema is not contagious, but the sores can become infected if not treated properly.	Inflamed skin One or a combination of rashes, pimples, scaly skin, and scabs The skin may be dry or have a watery discharge. The skin may itch or burn.	Soften crusts and dry skin with cold cream or oil. This often relieves itching. Prepare a lukewarm (39.6°C/98°F) bath for the child. Do not scrub the affected area with soap. Eczema can often be helped with drugs. But these drugs must be prescribed by a doctor.	Eczema may be caused by stress, or it may be an allergic reaction to something in the child's environment. It may also be a reaction to something in the child's diet in the previous two days. Eczema in babies is often related to milk allergies. This type of eczema does not respond to creams and does not heal easily.
Impetigo Bacterial Infection Contagious	Inflamed skin Clusters of pimples that: 1. become crusted and break, 2. are found around the mouth and nose, and 3. may be flat and pitted. They are filled with straw-coloured fluid.	Wash the infected area frequently with soap and water. Treat with saltwater solutions or antibiotics if prescribed by a doctor.	The most effective prevention for impetigo is careful handwashing by both the child and the caregivers. A child who has had impetigo should not return to the child care setting/school until prescribed medication has been taken for at least one full day.
Ringworm Fungal infection Contagious	Red, scaling rings on the skin	Clean the area twice a day with mild soap and water. After cleaning, apply prescribed anti-fungal ointment according to directions.	If the ringworm is extensive or if it persists even after treatment, the doctor may prescribe anti-fungal medication. A child who has had ringworm should not return to the child care setting/school until treatment has started.

Condition	What to Look For	🩹 What to Do	Remember
Scabies Skin parasite Contagious This is a reportable condition.	Many tiny blisters, scratch marks, and scaly crusts found mainly in skin folds (e.g., between fingers, on wrists, on the trunk, and on genitals) Extreme itchiness	Bathe in soap and water two nights in a row. Following the bath, apply the special lotion prescribed by the doctor.	Scabies is caused by the "itch mite." It burrows under the skin. To keep scabies from spreading, everyone in the household should be treated at the same time. After treatment, wash all bed linen, underclothes, and sleepwear. Wash blankets as well or press them with a hot iron. A child who has scabies should not return to the child care setting/school until treatment has been completed.
Prickly heat rash Not contagious	A rash of tiny, pin-point blisters surrounded by blotches of pink skin May appear on the face or on the parts of the body most heavily clothed. It occurs in hot weather or whenever the baby is overdressed.	If the baby is feverish, give her a sponge bath. Pat the baby's skin with cornstarch. Dress the baby more lightly and change her more frequently.	Prickly heat rash rarely bothers the baby, but if there is a fever at the same time, she may be irritable.
Diaper rash Not contagious	Red, scalded appearance that does not fade when left undiapered for a short period of time Pimples or sores found in the groin area	Wash and dry the area well. Expose the area to the air. Change diapers often. Use a zinc-based cream. If the rash does not clear up within 48 hours, seek medical attention.	Some diaper rashes are yeast infections. Watch for whitish, curd-like deposits found in genital folds that are not easily wiped away. May need to be treated with prescription ointment. A yeast infection can be contagious. Use proper precautions.

Condition	What to Look For	⚕ What to Do	Remember
Lice Contagious This is a reportable condition.	Small white eggs (nits) can be seen on the scalp, body hair, or pubic hair. They look like dandruff but cannot be washed off. Live lice may be seen. The scalp may show pustules and scabs due to scratching from extreme itchiness.	After the child has been seen by a public health nurse or doctor, use the appropriate medication. Shampoo the child's hair with soap and water. Then comb it with a fine-toothed comb to remove all the nits. Repeat the treatment as stated on the directions. All clothing and bedding that came into contact with the lice should be dry cleaned, washed in very hot water, or disinfected by freezing. Items such as stuffed animals or other items children sleep with, should be sealed in a plastic bag and kept out of reach for three weeks. The whole family may need to be treated. Vacuum the environment.	Lice are very common among children because children play close together. However, this is an extremely contagious condition and anyone can get it. It is more important to start treatment immediately than to worry about tracing the source. What to do to prevent lice: • Children's headgear should not be kept in a community box. • Hang hats on separate hooks. • Do not allow children to share combs. Lice are not caused by a lack of personal cleanliness. Children may return to the child care setting/school after the first treatment.
Pink eye Contagious	The white of the eye looks pink. Eyelids are usually swollen. Pus may form. Eyes are itchy or sensitive.	Protect the eyes from bright light. Do not let children share towels or washcloths. Pink eye should be reported to a doctor. The child should not rub or touch her eyes. Use warm water compresses on the eyes.	If the child's eyes have pus, keep her home from the child care setting/school until treated with warm water compresses and antibiotics for 24 hours. Pink eye is highly contagious; workers and family members need to follow the same rules as outlined for children.

Condition	What to Look For	What to Do	Remember
Pinworms Contagious	The child is constantly scratching around the anus. The child is unusually irritable. She may be awake and restless at night.	Make sure the child washes her hands using a nail brush. Keep the child's fingernails short. Discourage nail biting. Make sure the child has a daily bath or shower and a daily change of towels, sheets, and underwear. Prescription medication is usually needed. The whole family must be treated.	Pinworms are highly contagious. The child should therefore be kept home from the child care setting/school until after the first treatment dose. The medication is strongly coloured and will stain badly if the child spits it out.
Chicken pox Viral infection Contagious	Fever Rash, possibly with fluid-filled blisters Itchiness	The doctor may recommend a cream. Try to make sure the child does not scratch. Acetaminophen (e.g., Tylenol®) for fever (not acetylsalicylic acid—e.g., Aspirin®), as recommended by a doctor	Chicken pox is most contagious the day before the rash appears. Chicken pox can spread only through direct contact. The child should stay home if she has a fever or is not feeling well.
Diarrhea Underlying condition May be contagious	Unusually frequent, liquid bowel movements Blood in the stool Pain in the abdomen Other signs of illness Dehydration, which can be suspected if the child is passing less urine than usual	Seek medical attention for the following: • If there is blood in the stool • If the diarrhea is accompanied by vomiting • If it lasts for more than 72 hours Disinfect change area and toilet areas very carefully. Isolate a child who has severe diarrhea. Feed the child clear fluids for 24 hours. This means no fruit juice, soft drinks, or milk.	Diarrhea is a symptom of infection. It is caused by several kinds of germs. A child with very mild diarrhea may spread infection to someone else. Food poisoning or a change in diet can also cause diarrhea. Diarrhea is very common in children. For child care workers and babysitters: call parents/guardians if a child has diarrhea more than twice during the day.

Condition	What to Look For	✚ What to Do	Remember
		What to do if the child has two or more episodes of diarrhea: give special "rehydration" solutions as ordered by a doctor.	
Dehydration Not contagious	The child's diaper stays dry longer than usual or the child urinates less than the usual number of times in 8 to 10 hours. Dry mouth and tongue No tears when crying Sunken eyes In babies, the soft spot on the top of the head is sunken.	Seek medical attention. Continue to give fluids, as per a doctor's advice.	Dehydration results from a loss of body fluids. It is a serious risk, especially for babies, toddlers, and children. They can die if not treated quickly.
Ear aches	The child may be worried. She may pull at her ear or cover it with her hand. The child may complain of a sore ear. Fluid from the ear The child may develop fever, chill, deafness, dizziness, and nausea.	Seek medical attention. The infection may require an antibiotic.	
Persistent vomiting Underlying condition May be contagious	Nausea Stomach pain	Give the child only clear fluids. When the vomiting subsides, give small amounts of food, such as toast or diluted milk. If the vomiting continues, seek medical attention. If the vomiting is associated with diarrhea or pain, seek medical attention.	Persistent vomiting could be caused by illness, emotional upset, reaction to medication or a new food, or food poisoning.

FEVER

A fever by itself is not a reliable way to tell how sick a child is. A child may be very sick and not have a fever. On the other hand, a child might be running a fever and playing happily. The best indicator of illness is changes in behaviour.

> **NOTE:**
>
> *Normal body temperature is 37°C (or 98.6°F).*

 ## What to Do: Take the Child's Temperature

1 Wash your hands thoroughly.

2 Clean and reset the thermometer as per the manufacturer's guidelines.

3 Have the child sit in a comfortable place.

4 Make sure that the child has not had anything hot or cold to eat or drink in the past 10 minutes.

5 Take the child's temperature in one of the following areas:

- In the mouth, if the child is 4 years of age or older
- In the ear, if the child is 2 years of age or older

6 Leave the thermometer in place for as long as necessary to take the child's temperature. Check the manufacturer's guidelines.

> **NOTE:**
>
> *Taking the temperature in the armpit is not recommended.*

> **LOOK OUT FOR...**
>
> *Do not take the temperature rectally as this could cause damage to the bowel lining.*

7 Record the temperature, the time, and the method of taking the child's temperature.

 ## What to Do: Reducing a Child's High Fever

1 Sponge the child with water at room temperature. Make sure the child does not shiver.

2 Remove excess clothing and blankets.

3 Give the child water, diluted juice, or "flat" soft drinks.

> **NOTE:**
>
> *A fever shows that a body's defence mechanism is at work. A mild fever should not be a concern unless it continues for more than three days. If the child's temperature rises to 39°C (102°F) or if it is not easily controlled, seek medical attention.*

> **NOTE:**
>
> *Consult a doctor to determine what medication would be beneficial.*

▶ **Complications Related to Fever**

Reye's Syndrome

A child or teenager with a viral infection such as chicken pox or influenza may develop Reye's Syndrome if given ASA. Reye's Syndrome is a disease of the brain and liver that can lead to death. Consult your doctor.

Seizure

A baby or child may suffer a seizure when she has a high fever. (See Chapter 11 for what to do in the case of a seizure.)

GIVING MEDICATION

When to Give Medications

- Only with written permission from a parent or guardian for each day the medication is to be given
- Only with the written consent of a doctor (this applies to both prescription and nonprescription medications)
- Only when the medication is in the original container with the original label
- Only when the medication is properly labelled with:
  - ▶ The doctor's name
  - ▶ The child's name
  - ▶ The date the prescription was issued
  - ▶ The instructions
  - ▶ The time period during which the medication is to be taken

> **LOOK OUT FOR...**
>
> *If a child is being given non-prescription medications due to an illness, she is probably too ill to be attending the child care setting.*

How to Give Medications: General Rules

- Wash your hands thoroughly.
- Follow the "**Five Rights**":
  1. **Right medication**: Read the label when you are getting ready to give the medication.
  2. **Right amount**: Use an accurately marked measuring container.
  3. **Right time**: It is important to give medication at the right time.
  4. **Right child**: Make sure the child getting the medication is the one whose name is on the label of the medicine container.
  5. **Right method**: Read the directions carefully. Then give the medication correctly by mouth, by inhalation, through drops in the eyes, or through drops in the ears.

- Check the medication **three times**:
  1. When you take the medication from the cupboard or refrigerator
  2. When you take the medication out of the container, and
  3. Just before you administer the medication.

▶ How to Give Specific Medications

Medication in the Eye

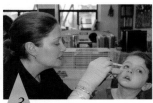

NOTE:
Use a separate cotton ball for each eye.

1 Have the child look up while in a lying or sitting position.

2 Gently pull down the lower eyelid.

3 Hold the dropper horizontally about one inch out from the child's eye.

4 Drop the medication into the little pocket between the lower lid and the eyeball.

5 Ask the child to close her eye. Then briefly hold a cotton ball against the inside corner of the eye.

6 Wipe away any excess medication.

Medication in the Nose

1 Have the child lie on a flat surface with her head hanging over one edge. If the child must sit up, have her tilt her head back as far as possible.

2 Place into each nostril the exact number of drops indicated in the prescription.

3 Have the child remain with her head back for a few minutes.

▶ Giving Medications

1. Keep a written record of the time the medication was given, the name of the child, the name of the medication, the person who gave the medication, and the amount given. Record all this information when you give the medication. This way the information will not be forgotten.

2. Call the parent or guardian if the child cannot keep the medication down.

3. Report to the parent or guardian or doctor any reactions or effects not usually experienced by the child.

NOTE:
Some provinces/territories have legislation regarding medication administration in child care settings. Please ask your Instructor for regulations in your area.

4. At the end of each day (or evening), tell the parent or guardian what medication was given and at what time.

5. Never dilute cough syrups.

6. Do not give medication in orange juice, milk, or any other essential food.

7. All the medication should be given for the recommended number of days.

8. Medicines that are no longer being used should be returned to the parent or guardian for disposal. Medications should be disposed of by returning them to a pharmacist

9. Store all medication out of the reach of children.

10. When applying ointments, protect yourself by using an applicator or by wearing disposable gloves.

11. When medications are being given for the first time, watch the child very closely for possible allergic reactions.

12. Medication, except for emergency medicines, should be locked up separately from the first aid kit.

13. Emergency medicine, such as inhalers or epinephrine auto-injectors, should be accessible at all times but out of reach of children.

CHILDHOOD CONDITIONS: GUIDELINES FOR CARE

1. Provincial or territorial legislation dictates which contagious diseases must be reported to the local health unit. Parents and guardians must also inform the local health unit, child care facility, and schools.

2. Take special precautions when attending to a child who has one of the conditions in Table 14.2, Childhood Conditions. For example, wear gloves and wash your hands frequently.

Keeping Children Safe

You are setting up a child care centre. Your centre will be accepting babies and children from three months of age and up. You need to purchase the necessary equipment and toys to accommodate babies, toddlers, and young children. You will need to consider what equipment and toys to purchase, as well as toys that are safe and age appropriate.

SAFE EQUIPMENT

Important:

- When considering second-hand equipment or toys, first check the label and contact Health Canada to find out if there are any safety issues related to that specific model.

- If the equipment or toys require repair, they will need to be thrown out or returned to the manufacturer to ensure their safety and that they continue to meet safety standards.

- Always have equipment and toys repaired professionally rather than attempt the repair yourself. Always follow the manufacturer's directions for safe use.

NOTE:

If you are having a safety problem with any product, you can contact Health Canada.

NOTE:

The Canadian Health Network (www.canadian-health-network.ca) is a wonderful resource for parents and caregivers. It includes information on a large number of topics, including keeping children safe and happy, what foods children should eat, and how children play and learn.

► Equipment for Babies

Safe Use of Cribs

- Cribs manufactured before September 1986 do not meet current safety standards and are best destroyed.

- Manufacturers of cribs are required to include a label showing the date of manufacture. If there is no label, assume that it is not safe.

- Allow only one small toy inside the crib and remove all mobiles or activity centres as soon as the baby can pull himself up.

- Be careful where you place a crib. It should be kept away from blind cords, windows, pictures, or shelves.

- When a child shows signs of trying to climb out of a crib, it is time to move him to a bed or mattress on the floor.
- Wheels on cribs should always be locked or removed once the child is able to pull up.
- Make sure that the crib slats are no more than 6 cm ($2^3/8$ in) apart.
- The height from the mattress support to the top rail must be at least 66 cm (2 ft, 2 in) when the support is in its lowest position.
- Make sure the mattress fits snugly inside the crib, as specified by Health Canada. Use only mattresses sold for use in cribs. Any other substitutes, such as foam pads, may allow for pockets or spaces in which a child may get stuck or smothered.
- Make sure that the corner posts extend no more than 3 cm ($1^1/4$ in) above the headboard and footboard.

Safe Use of Playpens

- Manufacturers of playpens are required to include a label showing the date of manufacture. If there is no label, assume that it is not safe.
- If a child shows signs of trying to climb out of a playpen, he is at risk of falling and it's time to store it away.
- Use playpens without wheels or with two wheels and two legs as opposed to a playpen with four wheels.
- Make sure that playpen walls are sturdy and at least 48 cm (1 ft, 7 in) high.
- Make sure hinges are designed and located to prevent pinching.

Safe Use of High Chairs

- Do not allow older children to climb on the chair. This holds true even when there is no baby or other child in the chair.
- A safe chair is stable and has a wide base to reduce the risk of tipping.
- The harness should consist of a strap that fits between the child's legs and a waist belt that is easy to fasten and kept in good condition.
- Ensure that the child's hands, arms, and legs are clear of any moving parts before making adjustments to the chair or the tray.
- Keep the chair a safe distance away from walls, doors, windows, blind cords, mirrors, appliances, and other furniture.

Safe Use of Baby Strollers

- Manufacturers of baby strollers are required to include a label showing the date of manufacture. If there is no label, assume that it is not safe.
- Do not load heavy parcels on the back or on the handles of the baby stroller. These could upset the stroller's balance.

- Use a stroller with a safety strap that goes around the child's waist and between the legs.
- Ensure children's fingers stay away from moving parts.

Safe Use of Pacifiers

- Before purchasing, make sure the pacifier is from a well-known manufacturer.
- Check pacifiers regularly for wear and tear. Discard immediately if there is any sign of deterioration, such as stickiness, discoloration, or hardening or cracking of the nipple.
- After a baby or child is diagnosed, by a doctor, with a yeast infection of the mouth, immediately discard any pacifier he is using. Give him a new one only after the infection has cleared.
- Changes in texture, tears, or holes can appear with age, heat, and exposure to food, sunlight, and medicine. For this reason, pacifiers should be changed at least every two months.
- Use a pacifier clip, as opposed to a cord, to secure the pacifier to the child.
- A teething ring should be used instead of a pacifier once the baby starts chewing.

Equipment for Children

Safe Use of Child Bike Trailers

LOOK OUT FOR...

Child carriers for bicycles can affect the steering and balance of the bicycle. The Canadian Paediatric Society considers them dangerous and therefore does not recommend them. A safer alternative to a child carrier is a child bike trailer.

Child bike trailers are recommended over child carriers because they reduce the risk of falls, do not cause as much of a steering or balance problem, and increase protection from the weather. They are also further from the bicycle wheel, ensuring that the child cannot reach the spokes.

- The best bike trailers have a five-point harness and roll bar.

- Attach a tall, bright flag to the trailer.
- The trailer should have a flexible joint so that if the bike tips, the trailer will not.
- As a bike trailer is wider than the bike, ensure that the wheels do not go over the road edge.
- Ride in low-traffic areas.
- Children should wear a properly fitting, approved helmet.

Safe Use of Safety Gates

- Manufacturers of safety gates are required to include a label showing the date of manufacture. If there is no label, assume that it is not safe.
- Supervise children carefully, even if a safety gate is in place.
- Use only approved safety gates. Avoid makeshift alternatives, such as a footstool or other object placed at the top or bottom of stairs.
- ALWAYS open and close gates to pass through. Climbing over a gate is unsafe and may cause an injury. It also models unsafe behaviour to children.
- Install safety gates wherever stairs are exposed. Make sure they are properly fitted and secure.
- If the gate has a pressure bar, make sure it is on the side away from children.
- If you can fit a pop can through household railings, a child could get stuck. To avoid this, cover the railings with rigid plastic or mesh.

SAFE USE OF TOYS FOR BABIES AND CHILDREN

- Follow the manufacturer's directions for safe use, including suggested age level. The Canadian Toy Testing Council issues a list of guidelines for choosing toys.
- When there are older siblings in the family, with toys that may have small parts, these toys should be separated and stored out of common play areas.
- Give children toys with rounded, smooth edges to prevent injury.
- Check batteries in toys regularly. Safely discard used batteries.
- Toys, paints, crayons, and markers must be completely washable and non-toxic.
- Provide only toys designed for babies or children. Giving them adult items such as wooden spoons or pots and pans to play with may seem safe but may present safety concerns. Many of these items are choking hazards, and if children think of them as toys, they might try to play with them at a time when they present a danger (e.g., when the same pot is full of hot water on the stove).
- Any plastic toys must be made of soft, bendable plastic because brittle plastic toys can be dangerous if broken.
- Ensure that toys and detachable pieces are too big to fit into a child's or baby's mouth, eyes, ears, or nose.

- Only provide toys without strings because strings may cause strangulation.
- Pull and tug on all parts of toys on a regular basis. If any parts detach, discard them. Discard the whole toy if you think it is unsafe. Look for cracks and loose pieces.
- Wooden toys should be glued or screwed together instead of nailed.
- Ride-around toys must be well balanced. Also, be sure to select them according to the size of the child.
- Children should wear helmets to suit the activity, such as regulation baseball, hockey, skateboarding, in-line skating, and bicycle helmets. "Toy" headgear is for imaginative play only.
- Electrical toys must bear the Canadian Standards Association (CSA) label. This confirms that they have been safety tested.
- Costumes must be made of flame-retardant materials. Use face paints instead of face masks to avoid blocking vision.
- Large toy boxes and other containers must have air holes and self-supporting hinges if it has a top. This is necessary in case children decide to hide inside. Allow children access only to boxes and other containers with loose-fitting lids or doors that have no locks.
- Children might consider old refrigerators or stoves to be a good place to hide or play in. It is important to keep these away from children and remove doors on old appliances so that children don't accidentally get locked inside.

▶ Extra Precautions for Babies

- Make sure that rattles and teethers are made of durable, smooth materials. Check labels to make sure that these materials are non-toxic.
- Make sure that mobiles are fastened securely and well out of the reach of babies.

PLAYING WITH TOYS SAFELY: SAFETY EDUCATION

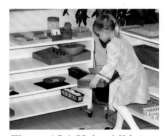

- Show children how to use toys.
- Some toys for older children are hazardous to younger children and babies. Help older children remember to keep these toys in their room with the door closed.
- To prevent tripping hazards, assign a toy box or special place for toys and help children remember to put toys away in these places (Figure 15.1).

Figure 15.1 Help children remember to put toys away.

SAFE USE OF PLAYGROUNDS

- Playgrounds are the sites of many serious injuries, mainly falls.
- Adults should always be present at playgrounds to supervise children. There should also be enough adults to properly watch all the children.
- Contact your local children's hospital, Health Canada, Safe Kids Canada, or your local/provincial/territorial injury prevention centre for information regarding playground safety or to obtain one of the safety checklists.

SAFE USE OF NEIGHBOURHOOD PLAYGROUNDS

Some public playgrounds are unsafe. Here are some safety considerations when checking out a playground (Figure 15.2):

- Examine park and school playgrounds for safety hazards.
- The most serious injuries result from falls onto hard surfaces.
- The best playground surfaces are loose sand, pine bark, and pea gravel 25 to 30 cm (10 to 12 in) deep.
- If you see unsafe or broken equipment in a playground, report this to the managing agency (e.g., community scentre, park board, school board).

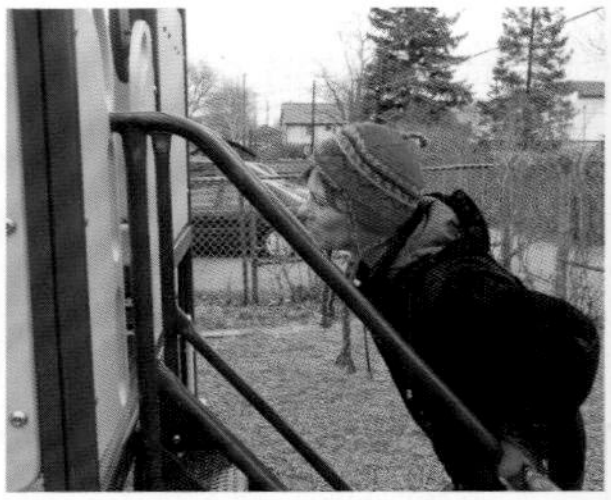

Figure 15.2 Ensure neighbourhood playgounds are safe.

SAFE USE OF BACKYARD PLAYGROUND EQUIPMENT

NOTE:

Provincial or territorial legislation specifies regulation for child care centre outdoor play equipment.

- Follow the playground equipment manufacturer's directions for safe installation, maintenance, use, and repair.
- When selecting playground equipment, consider the age and size of the children who will be using it.
- Check all equipment thoroughly and often using the following guidelines and any checklist provided by the manufacturer. All parts should be checked every two weeks.
- Make sure the following items are true for all backyard playgrounds:
  - ▶ Moving parts are covered to protect fingers and toes.
  - ▶ Swing seats are made of soft material, such as canvas or rubber.
  - ▶ Climbing equipment is designed to make it easy for children to climb down from it.

▶ Each sand box is fitted with a cover to keep dogs and cats from using it as a litter box.

▶ Only unleaded paint is to be used on playground equipment.

USING PLAYGROUNDS SAFELY: SAFETY EDUCATION

• Show children how to use equipment properly. Stop any dangerous behaviour immediately.

• Set and enforce a few simple rules for preventing injuries.

• Rules apply to all children, including visitors.

CAR SAFETY

NOTE:

*It is **against the law** to leave a baby or child alone in a car, even for a short time.*

Motor vehicle injuries are the number one cause of death of children in Canada. Follow the rules below to help ensure safety for children in and around motor vehicles.

SAFE USE OF CAR SEATS

It is required by law that all children use appropriate and approved child-restraint systems, such as infant or child seats and booster seats. These must have a label on them stating that they conform to the Canada Motor Vehicle Safety Standard, administered by Transport Canada.

• Children under the age of 12 should ride in the back seat.

• If you absolutely must put a child in the front seat of a car that has an airbag, push the seat back as far as it will go.

• No car seat should ever be put in the front seat.

• Manufacturers of car seats are required to include a label showing the model number and date of manufacture. When considering a second-hand car seat, first check the label and check with Transport Canada to see if there is a public notice on the seat. Discard the seat if it is more than 10 years old.

• Always follow the manufacturer's instructions for installation and use.

• Make sure that a child no longer in a car seat is secured with a seat belt. Show the child how to wear the belt. The lap belt should be low across the hips, and the shoulder belt should be over the shoulder and across the chest. If the seat belt does not fit properly, a booster seat should be used.

PASSENGER RULES FOR CHILDREN: SAFETY EDUCATION

Teach children the following rules for safety in and around motor vehicles:

- Always enter and exit the car on the curb side.

- Remain seated with your seat belt on while the car is moving. Stay that way until the car comes to a full stop.

- Remember that the driver needs to be able to concentrate on driving, not on distractions inside the car.

- Keep your head, arms, and feet in the car at all times.

- Remember that the car's controls are for the driver only. They're not for playing with, even when the car is parked.

> **NOTE:**
>
> *As a caregiver, ensure that everyone's fingers, hands, and feet are clear of doors before the doors are closed. Ensure that any person driving children has adequate insurance coverage.*

SAFE USE OF WHEELED EQUIPMENT

▶ Choosing a Safe Bicycle

- Make sure that the following are true for any bicycle used by a child:

  ▶ The bicycle is the proper size. Have the child stand over the bicycle with both feet flat on the ground. Lift the bicycle up to his body (both tires off the floor). There should be at least 2.5 cm (1 in) between the tires and the floor. When on the seat, the child should be able to put the balls of his feet on the ground.

  ▶ The brakes must work properly, and the child must be able to use them safely.

  ▶ Tires must be fully inflated.

  ▶ The wheels must be tightly secured and truly round.

  ▶ The chain must be oiled and tight.

  ▶ Spokes must be tight, straight, and unbroken.

  ▶ The bike must pass the "bounce test": the bike is bounced up and down on its wheels on the road while the adult listens for shakes and rattles. A safe bike is a quiet bike.

  ▶ The seat post and handlebars must be securely attached.

> **NOTE:**
>
> *Some local, provincial, or territorial legislation dictates that children must wear helmets.*

Choosing Safe Skateboards and In-line Skates (Rollerblades)

When choosing a skateboard or in-line skates, ensure that there are no loose or broken parts or sharp edges. Furthermore, a skateboard should not have a slippery top surface. Any defects should be repaired by a qualified repair person.

Choosing a Safe Helmet

> **NOTE:**
>
> *As a role model and for safety reasons, adults should always wear a helmet while riding a bicycle.*

Mishaps during sports requiring a helmet are the leading cause of head injuries for children in Canada. Wearing helmets can reduce the risk of a serious or fatal head injury by up to 80%.

- Use helmets approved by CSA (Canadian Standards Association), Snell, or ANSI (American National Standards Institute).

- A helmet should fit squarely on the child's head, with a snug chin strap.
- If the helmet is hit in a fall, buy another one. Even if the damage is not visible, it may have lost some of its ability to absorb shock.

Safe Use of Skateboards and In-line Skates (Rollerblades)

- Restrict skateboarding and in-line skating to children over five years of age.
- Allow children to use only playgrounds and paths built for skateboarding and in-line skating.
- Insist that children wear the correct equipment: a CSA-, Snell-, or ANSI-approved bicycle helmet, as well as elbow, wrist, and knee pads.

> **NOTE:**
>
> *Even the safest cyclist must watch for drivers who aren't paying attention!*

- Children should wear bright clothing while skateboarding or rollerblading. This way they will be visible to other people in the area and reduce the risk of collisions.

Safe Use of Bicycles

> **NOTE:**
>
> *Local legislation may dictate what needs to be on your bike for safety.*

- Walk bicycles across roads and streets only at intersections or pedestrian crosswalks.
- Before you cross, make sure that traffic crossing your path is fully stopped at stop signs or traffic signals.

- Ride in a straight line when you go down a road or street. Do not swerve between parked cars or onto driveways. Always look and signal in plenty of time before turning.
- Wear bright clothes even during the day. When motorists can see a cyclist, it's easier for them to co-operate with the cyclist.
- Children should not ride bicycles after dark.
- Bicycles should have a bell or horn.

> **NOTE:**
> *It is important to teach your children balancing, turning, hand signalling, and stopping on a bicycle before they go out riding. Practise these skills in the yard, a school yard, a park, or other low-traffic area.*

FIRE SAFETY

▶ Reducing the Risk of Fire and Burns

> **NOTE:**
> *For more information on reducing the risk of fire and burns, see Chapter 10 on burns.*

- Keep children away from heat sources and appliances such as cooking ovens, barbecues, space heaters, wood stoves, and fireplaces.
- Make sure all fireplaces and wood stoves are cleaned and inspected regularly to ensure that they follow safety codes.
- Space heaters must be at least 1 m (3 ft, 4 in) away from objects such as curtains and furniture.
- Turn pot handles in towards the centre of the stove.
- Keep cooking areas free of clutter. This will help prevent igniting pot holders, aprons, and other kitchen items.
- Snuff out candles immediately after use and keep all hot drinks out of children's reach.
- For nightwear, use only clothing designated as sleepwear. Other materials are sometimes more flammable. The government has set guidelines as to what is deemed sleepwear.
- Contact your local fire department for information on inspecting your home or workplace (including child care settings) for fire hazards and reviewing your fire escape plan.
- Make sure that smoke detectors are placed in all areas required by your local fire department or other agency that regulates fire safety in your area. Change the batteries in all smoke detectors twice a year.
- Keep bedroom doors or sleeping-area doors closed when children are sleeping. Doors are important barriers to smoke.
- Make sure that all breakers and fuses on the electrical panel in your home, workplace, or child care setting are clearly labelled.

- Use only single-cord plugs; multiple-cord or octopus plugs may over-heat. Keep loose cords secured and out of the way to prevent tripping and to keep children from pulling them out.
- Keep an approved, all-purpose chemical fire extinguisher in the kitchen.

Fire Escape Plan

Draw a floor plan. Mark the normal exit from each room. Then mark an emergency exit, such as a window. This exit can be used if fire blocks the doorway (Figure 15.3).

Identify a location where everyone will meet if they must escape from a fire. Check legislation as to how often this escape plan must be practised.

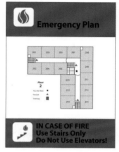

Figure 15.3 A fire escape plan for an apartment building.

What to Do in the Case of Fire During the Night

- When you hear the smoke detector, roll out of bed and onto the floor. Shout "Fire!"
- Crawl to the door and touch the door knob. If it is warm, do not open it. Unlock the door so that the firefighters can open it. Seal off any cracks with blankets or towels. Wet the blankets or towels if possible.

NOTE:

If a child spots a fire, he should know to shout, "Fire!" and get out of the building as quickly and safely as possible, and run to a spot where everyone has agreed to meet.

- Escape via the emergency exit. Be sure to practise this with children.
- If you cannot get out, take refuge in a room with a window. Open it for ventilation. Hang out a sheet as a signal for help.
- Decide who will assist those who cannot get themselves out, such as young children or someone with difficulty walking.
- Join everyone at the special meeting spot.

- After everyone is together, go to a neighbour's home to call the fire department.
- Meet the fire trucks and tell the firefighters that everyone has escaped the burning building.

IN CASE OF FIRE, SHOUT! THEN GET OUT!

ICE SAFETY

 ## Safe Skating or Walking on Ice

Teach children these safety rules for skating or walking on ice:

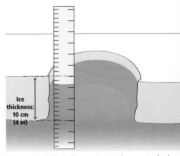

Figure 15.4 Ice must be a minimum of 10 cm (4 in) thick.

- Ice must be a minimum of 10 cm (4 in) thick before it can support one person (Figure 15.4). Ice must be solid and clear blue.

- Always skate with a buddy.

- When walking across unknown ice, carry a pole or hockey stick parallel to the ice surface.

If you fall through the ice:

- In shallow water, feel for the bottom with your feet. Then walk towards the shore or bank, breaking ice as you go. Keep going until you can slide up onto thicker ice.

- In deep water, flutter-kick your feet and extend your hands forward along the ice until you can slide up onto it. Slowly crawl to safety.

- After you are out of danger, get to shelter and change into warm clothing. This will help prevent hypothermia.

SAFE USE OF WATER

 ## Safe Use of Bathtubs

- Always be present when a baby or child is in a bathtub or bathing basin. Drowning can occur even in a few centimetres of water.

- Check bathwater temperature by splashing water on your inner wrist. If this feels too hot or cold to you, do not place the baby or child in the bath.

- If your bathtub is a Jacuzzi type or is equipped with water jets, refrain from turning these on with the baby or child in the tub.

- Turn off all water taps tightly.

- Install protective covers over faucets to prevent injury should anyone slip and fall against them while in the tub.

 ## Safe Use of Backyard Pools and Hot Tubs

- Keep children under constant supervision when they are playing in or around a backyard pool or hot tub.

- Make sure basic lifesaving equipment is available at all times. Examples of basic lifesaving equipment are (1) a strong, lightweight pole with blunt ends and (2) a ring buoy with a long throwing rope. Be aware of pool safety equipment requirements outlined in the legislation governing your area.

- Cover hot tubs securely and lock them when they are not in use.
- Keep decks around the pool or hot tub clean and free of debris.
- Pay close attention to the surface of the diving board. Make sure the slip-resistant surface is always in good repair.
- Use only unbreakable cups, dishes, and other utensils at the poolside.
- Keep electrical appliances away from a backyard pool.
- Remove all floating toys when pool time is over.
- Install a lifeline across the pool where the deep end slope begins.
- Make sure electrical equipment used to operate the pool or hot tub conforms to electrical code requirements.
- Install a phone on the pool deck. Post a list of emergency numbers beside it.
- Ensure that an outdoor pool is surrounded by a fence, wall, building, or enclosure that children cannot get through or over. These protections must conform to fencing requirements for your local municipality. Gates should have self-closing latches above the reach of toddlers. They should also include hardware for permanent locking.
- Make sure all pool chemicals are stored in a secure area.

▶ Safe Swimming

- Make sure that children and adults learn to swim. Take Canadian Red Cross swimming lessons.
- Ensure children are always supervised by an adult. Children should keep away from unsupervised bodies of water.
- Establish sensible safety rules before children do any swimming. Enforce these rules consistently and firmly.
- Swimmers must always swim with a buddy. Sudden cramps can sink the most accomplished swimmer.
- Allow swimming only in good weather, during daylight.
- Nonswimmers and those supervising them need to realize the dangers of using inner tubes or air mattresses in the water.
- Always stay within specified boundaries.
- When distance swimming at the beach, make sure that children swim parallel to shore.
- Always know the depth of the water and ensure it is clear of all obstacles before diving.
- Post "No Diving" signs around above-ground pools.
- Allow only one person at a time on diving boards or water slides.
- Swimmers must stay away from the area underneath diving boards.

Safe Boating

- Make sure that all boat occupants are wearing approved life jackets or approved personal flotation devices (PFDs). Look for PFDs with labels stating that they have been approved by Transport Canada, the Canadian Coast Guard, or Fisheries and Oceans Canada.

- As a parent or caregiver of a child, set a good example by wearing your life jacket or PFD and by following boating safety rules.

- Small crafts can be unstable. Teach children to stay low in the boat.

- Teach children how to use a boat radio and fire extinguisher in case of an emergency.

- Discuss and practise survival techniques often.

- Choose both PFDs and life jackets carefully to match the wearer's size and weight.

- Children should use PFDs fitted with crotch straps. The strap must be used when wearing the PFD.

- All pleasure crafts, power vessels, sailing vessels, canoes, kayaks, and rowboats must carry safety equipment in good working order. To find out exactly what is needed for your boat, contact Transport Canada.

- As of September 15, 2009, anyone operating a powerboat on Canadian waters must have a pleasure craft operator card. Contact your local Canadian Red Cross office for more information on where to obtain your certification.

BABYSITTERS

Choose babysitters who demonstrate knowledge of injury prevention. They should have taken first aid training or a babysitting course that includes first aid. The Canadian Red Cross Society offers these types of courses. To learn more about these courses, visit www.redcross.ca or call 1-877-356-3226.

TEACHING CHILDREN SAFETY AWARENESS

Teach children how to get help in an emergency:

- Teach them to go to a trusted neighbour.
- Teach them about the Block Parent Program of Canada in your area, if applicable.
- Make a list of emergency phone numbers and teach children what to say when they call EMS/9-1-1:

▶ Their name

▶ The address they are calling from

▶ What the problem is

▶ The number they are calling from

• Teach children to "hang up last" when they call EMS/9-1-1. This way the dispatcher will have all the necessary information.

• Teach children about traffic safety.

CHILD AND YOUTH PROTECTION

There are different types of abuse. It is important to be able to understand the different situations in which abuse towards children and youth may occur. Many of these situations are preventable, and if you are able to recognize the signs, you may be able to intervene on a child's or youth's behalf.

Vulnerable Children and Youth

All children and youth live with some risk of experiencing abuse, violence, neglect, and bullying or harassment.

Abuse and Violence

Abuse and violence may take different forms: emotional, physical, and sexual.

Emotional abuse is defined as a CHRONIC attack on a child's or youth's self-esteem.

Physical abuse is when a person in a position of power or trust purposefully injures or threatens to injure a child or youth.

Sexual abuse occurs when a younger or less powerful child is used by an older or more powerful child, adolescent, or adult for sexual gratification.

Neglect

Neglect is the CHRONIC inattention to the basic necessities of life, such as clothing, shelter, nutritious diet, education, good hygiene, supervision, medical and dental care, adequate rest, a safe environment, moral guidance and discipline, exercise, and fresh air.

▶ Understanding Bullying and Harassment

Bullying

Bullying involves a person expressing his power through the humiliation of another person.

Types of Bullying

- **Physical:** hitting or kicking victims or taking or damaging property
- **Verbal:** name-calling, insults, negative comments, and constant teasing
- **Relational:** trying to cut victims off from social connection by convincing peers to exclude or reject the victim; most common among girls
- **Reactive:** engaging in bullying, as well as provoking bullies into attacking them by taunting

Harassment

According to the Canadian Human Rights Commission, *discrimination* is treating people "differently, negatively or adversely" on the basis of a prohibited ground of discrimination under federal, provincial, or territorial human rights legislation (2005).

Types of Harassment

- **Personal:** based on an individual's personal characteristics that are prohibited grounds for discrimination
- **Racism:** when people are treated negatively because of their colour or racial or ethnic background
- **Sexual harassment:** unwelcome behaviour of a sexual or gender nature that negatively affects the person or the environment
- **Criminal harassment:** when the harassing behaviour contravenes Canada's Criminal Code

▶ Responding to Abuse, Bullying, and Harassment

Verbal Disclosures

When children or youth make a verbal disclosure about abuse, bullying, or harassment, it is important to follow the **HEARD** procedure:

H Hear and honour the youth and the information.

E Empathize and encourage.

A Affirm the youth. Acknowledge choices.

R Report/refer. Respond to organizational policies.

D Document accurately. Determine care of self.

Handling a Spoken Disclosure from a Child or Youth

1. Listen calmly and openly:
   - As the child speaks, you may be overrun with your own feelings of anger, pain, and perhaps fear.
   - Be emotionally available to the child and listen.
   - Do not ask questions; do not interview.
   - Do not make judgments about the child or possible abuser.
   - Give full attention to the child and nod understandingly as the story comes out.
   - To ensure that the child's message is not overheard by others, move away from onlookers.
   - If you are inside, find a room that is neutral to both the child and you, where you have privacy, but always leave the door slightly open.

2. Reassure:
   - As a responsible adult in a position of trust, you must believe that this child has come to you with something to tell because of powerful, hurtful feelings.
   - Trust that the child is speaking from great need and open your heart to hear.
   - Children who speak about sexual, physical, or emotional abuse often struggle with the desire to protect the abuser.

Nonverbal Disclosures

When abuse, bullying, or harassment is suspected, the procedure for responding to a nonverbal disclosure is **DARE**:

D Document accurately.

A Affirm the information. Acknowledge and affirm the child or youth. Acknowledge choices.

R Report/refer. Respond to organizational polices.

E Establish accurate records. Execute care of self.

For more information on child and youth protection or to take a RespectED course, please visit our Website at www.redcross.ca.

First Aid Supplies

A first aid kit for home use should contain the following. Remember to replenish and maintain contents on a continuing basis.

1. Emergency telephone numbers for EMS/9-1-1, the local Poison Control Centre, and personal doctors. Include the home and workplace phone numbers of family members, friends, and neighbours who can help.

2. Sterile gauze pads (dressings) in small and large squares to place over wounds

3. Adhesive tape

4. Roller and triangular bandages to hold dressings in place or to make an arm sling

5. Adhesive bandages in assorted sizes

6. Scissors

7. Tweezers

8. Safety pins

9. Ice bag or chemical ice pack

10. Disposable gloves such as surgical or examination gloves (non-latex, non-vinyl)

11. Flashlight, with extra batteries in a separate bag

12. Antiseptic wipes or soap

13. Pencil and pad

14. Emergency blanket

15. Eye patches

16. Thermometer for taking the child's temperature

17. Pocket mask or barrier device

18. Canadian Red Cross *Child Care First Aid & CPR Manual*

Personal Emergency Information

Child's Name _____

Date of Birth _____

Child's Health Card Number _____

Parent or Guardian's Name, Address, and Telephone Number(s) _____

_____

_____

_____

_____

Paediatrician

   Name _____

   Telephone Number(s) _____

Family Doctor

   Name _____

   Telephone Number(s) _____

Medical Specialist(s)

   Name _____

   Telephone Number(s) _____

Dentist

    Name _____

    Telephone Number(s) _____

Medical Insurance

    Name of Company _____

    Policy Number_____

    Company's Telephone Number(s)_____

Allergies _____

_____

Chronic Conditions _____

_____

Special Information and Precautions _____

_____

_____

_____

_____